A GOOD DEATH:
ON THE VALUE OF
DEATH AND DYING

FACING DEATH

Series editor: David Clark, Professor of Medical Sociology
University of Lancaster

The subject of death in late modern culture has become a rich field of theoretical, clinical and policy interest. Widely regarded as a taboo until recent times, death now engages a growing interest among social scientists, practitioners and those responsible for the organization and delivery of human services. Indeed, how we die has become a powerful commentary on how we live and the specialized care of dying people holds an important place within modern health and social care.

This series captures such developments. Among the contributors are leading experts in death studies, from sociology, anthropology, social psychology, ethics, nursing, medicine and pastoral care. A particular feature of the series is its attention to the developing field of palliative care, viewed from the perspectives of practitioners, planners and policy analysts; here several authors adopt a multi-disciplinary approach, drawing on recent research, policy and organizational commentary, and reviews of evidence-based practice. Written in a clear, accessible style, the entire series will be essential reading for students of death, dying and bereavement, and for anyone with an involvement in palliative care research, service delivery or policy-making.

Current and forthcoming titles:

David Clark, Jo Hockley and Sam Ahmedzai (eds): *New Themes in Palliative Care*
David Clark and Jane E. Seymour: *Reflections on Palliative Care*
David Clark and Michael Wright: *Transitions in End of Life Care: Hospice and Related Developments in Eastern Europe and Central Asia*
Mark Cobb: *The Dying Soul: Spiritual Care at the End of Life*
Kirsten Costain Schou and Jenny Hewison: *Experiencing Cancer: Quality of Life in Treatment*
David Field, David Clark, Jessica Corner and Carol Davis (eds): *Researching Palliative Care*
Anne Grinyer: *Cancer in Young Adults: Through Parents' Eyes*
Henk ten Have and David Clark (eds): *The Ethics of Palliative Care: European Perspectives*
Jenny Hockey, Jeanne Katz and Neil Small (eds): *Grief, Mourning and Death Ritual*
Jo Hockley and David Clark (eds): *Palliative Care for Older People in Care Homes*
David W. Kissane and Sidney Bloch: *Family Focused Grief Therapy*
Gordon Riches and Pam Dawson: *An Intimate Loneliness: Supporting Bereaved Parents and Siblings*
Lars Sandman: *A Good Death: On the Value of Death and Dying*
Jane E. Seymour: *Critical Moments: Death and Dying in Intensive Care*
Anne-Mei The: *Palliative Care and Communication: Experiences in the Clinic*
Tony Walter: *On Bereavement: The Culture of Grief*
Simon Woods: *Death's Dominion: Ethics at the End of Life*

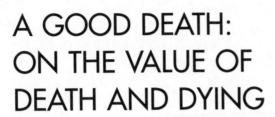

A GOOD DEATH:
ON THE VALUE OF
DEATH AND DYING

LARS SANDMAN

OPEN UNIVERSITY PRESS

Open University Press
McGraw-Hill Education
McGraw-Hill House
Shoppenhangers Road
Maidenhead
Berkshire
England
SL6 2QL

email: enquiries@openup.co.uk
world wide web: www.openup.co.uk

and Two Penn Plaza, New York, NY 10121–2289, USA

First published 2005

A catalogue record of this book is available from the British Library

ISBN 0335 21411 8 (pb) 0335 21412 6 (hb)

Library of Congress Cataloging-in-Publication Data
CIP data applied for

Typeset by RefineCatch Ltd, Bungay, Suffolk
Printed in the UK by MPG Books, Bodmin

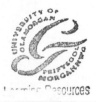

Contents

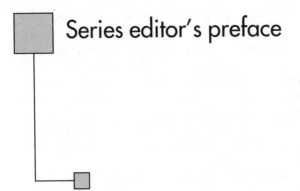

Series editor's preface

One of the features of the modern palliative care specialty is the rather overt normative and ideological value system that accompanies it. The practitioners and proponents of palliative care have not been shy in propounding what is best for patients and families at the end of life. Of course, much of this has been couched in a language concerned to promote the interests of patients and families and which gives an important place to the concept of autonomy as well as to respecting choices, beliefs and preferences. It might also be said that this normative confidence has been a key to the success of palliative care development – leading to service innovation, policy recognition, and financial reimbursement. But as the field matures it is important and necessary to subject such values to close scrutiny, particularly from disciplines with the analytic power and the resources to make sense of what is happening when palliative care impacts upon the world. That is what makes this book so important..

Lars Sandman is a Swedish philosopher with expertise in ethics and an interest in palliative care. He has written a book for the Facing Death series that builds on some of the debates identified by other volumes in the series. He was a participant in the well-known *Pallium* project that was brought together in an edited collection entitled *The Ethics of Palliative Care*[1] and he addresses concerns that have been explored in *Reflections on Palliative Care*[2] as well as in the ethnographic studies we have published by Jane Seymour[3] and Anne Mei The[4]. But in his own analysis he goes well beyond these to offer us a full-blown exploration of the value systems at work in palliative care as it seeks to serve patients facing death and those close to them.

What is at the heart of his argument?

Sandman adopts a consequentialist position, so he is interested in the effects which actions and interventions have on those involved. He presents a 'birds eye' view of the palliative care system in which *all* the actors appear in a moral universe of complex inter-connection. This allows him to take account of the specific circumstances of patients, close ones and carers. It also gives a place to wider structural factors that might shape the context of giving and receiving care at the end of life. Most importantly of all, he is interested in how we make sense of the process of giving value to life, and sees this as the starting point to how we might think about care when life is ending and a 'good death' is sought.

Is a 'good death' one which is morally consistent with the life that has preceded it? How might we characterise a meaningful death? And what is meant by a dignified death? Sandman takes up each of these questions in turn, but is left doubting the necessity of any of them as essential elements within a global schema of the 'good death'. Likewise he explores through a number of examples whether we have reason to face death in a specific way: acquainted with it through the death of others; aware of our own situation; accepting the end of life; in control of our emotional responses; and with our suffering controlled. Again he can find no logical argument for a normative rule to guide us on any of these dimensions. Nor can he identify compelling reasons to make a stand on behalf of any of the various preparations for death that are variously promoted in modern palliative care: ritual observances; completion of worldly affairs; end of life review; and staging one's departure in a modern ars moriendi. He also finds arguments which try to show the importance of peace and tranquillity at the end of life, or the necessary presence of close ones at a death, or the absence of technology when a person dies – all to be largely unconvincing.

This amounts to an important appraisal in which each well known element generally considered vital to a 'good death' in palliative care is held up to close scrutiny. In so doing, Sandman shows that in every case it is possible for 'good death' to take place in a contrary fashion. The importance for practice becomes strikingly clear. For Sandman, the *only* route to the good death is that chosen (explicitly or implicitly) by the individual dying person. Promoting the 'good death' is therefore about respecting autonomy and the goals of the patient – however engaged or disinterested they may be in the details.

I believe this book will be welcomed by modern practitioners of palliative care. It provides further strength to the argument for individualising the goals of care at the end of life. In particular, it emphasises that care of a person in the final months, weeks and days, cannot be detached from the whole life that has gone before. Sandman makes it clear that palliative care can have an important role in adding value to the process of dying, but it can only do so by applying the strictest discipline of patient-centredness and respect for autonomy. At the same time palliative carers have an obligation to help guide patients towards their desired goals, through careful use of their professional training and expertise. There is a fine line to be walked here between assuming that the patient's autonomy can be exercised at all times, and eroding autonomy through the professional framing of a particular sort of 'good death'. Those carers who read this thoughtful and humane analysis may well emerge better equipped to maintain a balance between the two.

David Clark

References

1 Ten Have, H. and Clark, D. (2002) *The Ethics of Palliative Care: European Perspectives*. Buckingham: Open University Press.
2 Clark, D. and Seymour, J. (1999) *Reflections on Palliative Care*. Buckingham: Open University Press, pp. vii–viii.
3 Seymour, J.E. (2001) *Critical Moments: Death and Dying in Intensive Care*. Buckingham: Open University Press.
4 The, A.M. (2002) *Palliative Care and Communication: Experiences in the Clinic*. Buckingham: Open University Press.

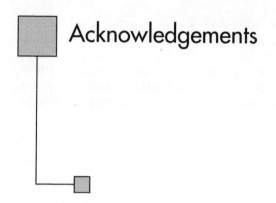

Acknowledgements

This book is an abridged and revised version of my doctoral dissertation (with the same title) and hence I am greatly indebted to my supervisor for enabling me to write the original document, on which this book is based, Professor Torbjörn Tännsjö. I am also indebted to a former collegue of mine who also commented extensively on the original thesis, Docent Christian Munthe, and to all others who took part in the seminars at the Philosophy Department, Gothenburg University, Sweden.

I would also like to express my sincere gratitude to Professor David Clark both for enabling me to be a part of the Facing Death series and for commenting on earlier drafts of the manuscript and bringing my attention to a large section of social science literature formerly uncovered by me. Even though, evidently, there is plenty more left where that came from.

Furthermore, I would like to thank Dr Simon Woods for providing me with a manual for how to write a good book outline to the publishers and for giving me good references. And I would also like to thank all the people at Open University Press/McGraw-Hill who have been supportive and encouraging during the process, especially Rachel Gear, and the Department of Caring Sciences, University College of Borås, Sweden, for giving me some time to write the book.

Last, but not least, I am always indebted to my family for putting up with my, not always day-scheduled, work.

However much indebted to others, I am of course fully responsible for the discussion and conclusions of this book.

Introduction

This book is not written out of a morbid interest in death and dying. On the contrary, I seldom give death and dying much thought in my private life. A personal motive for writing this book is that I have been provoked by the many ideas on how to achieve a good death found when doing research in palliative care – ideas claiming that we should adopt certain attitudes and make certain preparations, or that death should have certain features in order for us to arrive at a good death. Hence a fundamental question for this book is whether we have good reasons to adopt these attitudes or make these preparations, or for death to have these features – in the sense that doing so will do us good.

However, the main reason for writing this book is not my own indignation but the fact that ideas on good death seem to play an important normative role within palliative care and might affect what attitude carers adopt towards dying people and what care dying people will be provided with; a problem of greater dignity rather than my own indignation or aggravation. In Walter (1994) it is argued that there is a conflict between the overall norm about allowing patients to die in whatever way they like found within palliative care, and some of the more specific views on what is the best way, also part of palliative care. I do find this overall norm to be a good norm in our pluralistic society and hence want to take a closer critical look at some of these more specific views that might influence people to die in a way that is not of their own choice.

This also implies that the discussion is focused on a good dying in distinction from the more encompassing concept of good death, which relates to the period of dying, the event of death, and what happens after death (Momeyer 1988). Henceforth, I will mainly be talking in terms of a good dying.

In effect, in this book I try to show the complexity of the question of a good dying and the extent to which we need to be careful in passing judgement on what a good dying is for particular individuals – since they might have good reasons to want to deviate from what *we* consider to be a good dying. The discussion shows that these notions of dying:

- add differently to the value of our lives depending on what theory of value we accept;
- have supporting as well as undermining reasons to go with them even given the same value theory;
- to a large extent depend on the individual context of the dying in question.

Given the above, it seems that we should be careful in making universal claims about the goodness of dying.

The choice of ideas on good dying discussed in this context is limited to ideas from a modern Western context and in particular from the context of modern Western palliative care (henceforth just palliative care). Obviously there are a large number of ideas on good dying not explicitly dealt with in this context, especially those closely associated with religious or cultural world-views other than the ones influencing palliative care. I tend to agree with those who claim that ideas about good death are, in a lot of cases, closely associated with religious and cultural ideas about an afterlife or a transcendent reality (see, for example, De Marinis 1998; Walter 2003). Still, the focus of the book is the good dying advocated within palliative care, and a discussion of further ideas would bring us too far away from this focus.

It has been argued that most of the ideas discussed in this context (i.e. most or all of the ideas found within palliative care) fit very well with the (modern or postmodern) value of individual control and of people fashioning their lives for themselves as they see fit, not following or adhering to any traditions or overall formulas for how to live one's life (in Walter 1994; Seale 1998; Smith 2000; Clark 2003, discussing a good death, the emphasis is on patients' control over their dying and death). I find this rather convincing and, given this, the ideas on good dying found in this context could be questioned following a questioning of such a value or view of people, as Walter, Seale and others to some extent seem to do. However, I have chosen a somewhat different perspective in this book, in accepting that a lot of Western people have an interest in fashioning a good life for themselves and their close ones (even if not necessarily through the kind of control advocated in palliative care) and in taking a look at the ideas of good dying to see whether they could actually bring about such a good life at the end of life.

As indicated, besides discussing different ideas on a good dying I will also try to indicate something about how the conclusions of the discussion might affect the practice of palliative care. In the final chapter of the book I say something general about what role ideas on good dying could and should have within palliative care. More generally, I continually return to the normative aspects of different ideas, with a short concluding comment following the idea on good dying discussed. To enable the reader to follow the discussion of the book I start with a short introduction to the perspective on ethics and value used in the book. I also say something about the relationship between dying, death and post-death and about the value of the event of death. The latter might in many cases be relevant to the discussion of a good dying.

The main part of the book is dedicated to the discussion of a number of different ideas on good dying, grouped under four headings: 'Global features of death and dying', 'Facing death', 'Prepared to die' and 'The environment of dying and death'.

Generally, the ideas on good dying and death are discussed according to the following structure. First, I outline different possible interpretations of the idea that are relevant in this context. Second, I discuss what value following the idea would have to the dying patient. Third, I discuss whether there are any specific problems affecting the lives of close ones and carers in relation to the idea. Finally, I discuss whether there are any specific normative considerations to take into account in relation to the idea. Here, the comments in relation to the ideas presented earlier will be somewhat more extensive, so that, to the extent that they are generalizable to the following ideas, they will not be repeated. Since the focus of the book is on different reasons for the value of specific ideas on good dying and death, the normative comments are rather short and should only be taken to indicate a sense of normative direction in how to think about individual cases, not as absolute recommendations or rules.

1 Ethics and value

In order to discuss whether a certain action or attitude leads to a good or better death we need a few tools. First, we need to have some idea about what it is that generally contributes to the good of a human life, i.e. we need to have some kind of hunch about value theory. Some general ideas on value theory are presented below. However, even if we have good reasons to believe that a certain action leads to a better death, it is not thereby evident that we should actually perform the action or that it is ethically required or allowed or has anything to do with ethics at all. This will depend on what kind of ethical perspective or theory we adopt. For example, if we have a so-called deontological perspective on ethics regulating that certain type of actions should be done or not done, due to their internal characteristics and not due to their consequences, the value of what we do will be of less import-ance. According to such a theory we should, for example, abstain from lying even if we thereby cause the world to be worse, value-wise. From such a perspective the value discussion of this book will not be ethically relevant to a large extent. It will be relevant from a so-called prudential perspective, i.e. to the extent we want to live and die good lives and deaths. However, the ethical perspective adopted in this book is not deontological but consequen-tial and from such a perspective it is essential what outcome our actions will bring along. Hence, in the first section of this chapter I briefly present the ethical perspective or theory adopted in the discussion of this book.

Ethical perspective

The discussion in this book rests on the assumption that when we try to find out what we should (ethically) do in a situation of care, we need to know how the different alternatives add to the value of people's lives. In effect, the ethical perspective from which the book is written assumes that the consequences of our actions and attitudes are the single most important factor deciding whether we should do these actions or have these attitudes, i.e. it is consequentialistic in its approach.

This is not the place nor is there the space to defend a fully fledged version of consequentialism (see, for example, Smart and Williams 1973, Tännsjö 1998a, for a discussion of consequentialism), and hence I boldly assume that the consequences of what we do are of central importance to ethics. If so, the discussion of the value that different actions and attitudes in relation to death will bring about is going to be ethically relevant. However, since the comments in the sections termed 'Normative aspects of . . .' assume this consequentialistic approach, I will elaborate somewhat more on this perspective. First, the term 'normative' relates to the fact that 'normative ethics' is the branch of ethics dealing with theories and criteria for how to solve practical ethical problems. Hence, when we talk in terms of normative aspects or normative claims, it implies that we are saying something about what the discussion of value should imply for what we should do in relation to dying patients and their close ones.

When judging what to do in a situation of care from a consequentialistic perspective, we will have to take all consequences into consideration. Hence, we will have to take all involved parties into consideration, i.e. the dying patient, his or her close ones and the care personnel, since they are all likely to be affected by what we do. However, we will also have to keep an eye on what would happen in a greater perspective, i.e. what would happen to people outside the care context if we chose a certain alternative. For example, in relation to the discussion on euthanasia it has been argued that even if we find it the best possible action in the care situation to actively and intentionally cause a person to die, we should be aware of what could happen at a societal level if we allow people to be actively and intentionally killed within the health-care system.

At the same time, even if we should judge what to do from the actual consequences that will result in the situation at hand, it seems that we should accept certain restrictions on what to do: restrictions that can be supported by consequentialistic reasons as being the best strategy in the long run. First, we should be extremely wary of disrespecting the self-determination of the patient or close one. That is, if we judge that some course of action would benefit the patient or close one we should (normally) still respect their decision, even if it goes against what we judge as beneficial. Only in special cases could we go against the will of the patient or close one – for example, when the course of action will be seriously harmful to someone else or when we have very good reasons to believe that the course of action chosen by the patient or close ones is not really what they want.

Second, we should distribute the goods we can provide within the health-care system in a just way, where 'the goods' are here understood in terms of the value we might add to people's lives. Hence, if we can contribute to the good life or death of a patient or close one we should do so, as long as this does not prevent us from benefiting other people within our care to a reasonably similar degree.

Third, care personnel cannot be required to provide care that goes beyond their role as care professionals. For example, even if a close and intimate relationship is what would be in the patient's best interest, the care professional cannot be required to enter into such a relationship with the patient. That is, even if palliative carers sometimes portray themselves as more than professional carers (see, for example, Lawton 2000) it will here be assumed that palliative carers cannot ethically be made to do more than what is within their role as professional carers; though, of course, they may do so voluntarily.

These restrictions or side-constraints will be taken for granted in the discussion and not explicitly referred to unless there are special considerations to address concerning them in relation to a certain idea.

Another aspect of consequentialism is that we need to look at other factors besides what carers or others do that might influence the outcome of care. For example, we need to look at how structural factors might influence the possibility of adding value to dying persons' lives, i.e. factors like the judicial situation, the economic situation, the organizational structure, leadership, routines, care culture and other structural factors. However, this is something that to a large extent lies outside the explicit discussion of this book, and I comment only on the aspect of care culture.

Before moving over to different ideas about what characteristics the consequences we are trying to achieve should have, i.e. ideas about what adds value to a human life, we should say something about the extent to which dying persons have moral responsibilities when at the end of their lives. This is relevant to situations when the good of the dying person and the good of close ones seem to conflict. Weisman (1972: 36) has claimed that making moral demands on a dying person could be viewed as 'sanctimonious cruelty' (see also Momeyer 1988: Chapter 6). However, I see no reason to give a dying person moral leeway when at the end of life. It is important to remember that even the dying person can act in a morally problematic way (Ellingson and Fuller 1998). However, I do find it reasonable to lower our moral demands on him or her, simply because of the lack of strength and functions of such a person and not due to the fact that he or she is dying. That is, part of being a human person is to be someone who has moral responsibilities and of whom one can make moral demands, and it would seem to emphasize the depersonalization dying might result in to give dying persons moral leeway (see the discussion on depersonalization found in Lawton 2000).

Value theory or something about the good of life

In order to be able to work out the best possible consequences of an action or attitude we will need an idea about what is best or good, i.e. we need to have an idea about what might add to the value of people's lives. Hence, in this section there is a brief exposition of central theories on value found in philosophical and ethical discussions. Before moving on to a presentation of different theories about what contributes to a good life, i.e. what has value, we need to say something about the distinction between instrumental and final value in relation to the project of this book.

When looking at a specific idea about good dying we need to know whether the feature found in this idea is valuable as an end; or as a means to an end; or, in the above terminology, whether it has final or instrumental value. The reason for this is that the instrumental value of a certain feature will depend on whether that which it furthers (if it so does) is valuable and if so finally valuable, or if we need to move even further on this means–end trajectory.

In the medieval *Ars Moriendi* tradition[1] one of the features of a good death was to review one's life when on the death bed and the main reason for such a review was that it enabled you to repent and hence prepare for a future life in heaven. In other words, the review was instrumentally important in relation to the probably final value of blissful existence in heaven. However, nowadays we might not be as convinced about the existence of places like heaven and hell. With the disappearance of heaven we seem to have lost the final value to be pursued in making a life review. Still, we might find other ways of justifying the practice, since bliss in heaven might not be the only final value it furthers. On the other hand, if we do not find any final values that it furthers it seems that we will have to give up our claims concerning the goodness of reviewing.

In the end, therefore, our ideas about good death must rest on some notion of what is valuable as an end or in itself, i.e. finally valuable. This motivates a brief exposition of standard theories on final value. In the philosophical literature (see, for example, Parfit 1984: 3ff; Griffin 1996; Brülde 1998) we find three different versions of what is good for persons: hedonistic theory, desire fulfilment theory and objective list theory. In this context I will take as a starting point that there is something to all these theories and that we might accept a complex theory of a good life. This means I will use them in the following manner in the discussion. I will take it that hedonism or experiential well-being is at the heart of a good life and something we will judge as central in many situations. However, I will also take it that sometimes we might have reasons to act in discord with our well-being, since there are other, non-hedonistic aspects of a good life that might motivate this. Hence, when desire fulfilment theory will give us more general reasons to act against our well-being or when there is some item on the objective list that will give us such a reason, I will bring them into the discussion.

Hedonistic theory

Classically, hedonistic theory has been formulated in terms of pleasure and pain, where only the person's own experiences of pleasure can be good as an end for this person and only the person's own experiences of pain or suffering or displeasure can be bad as an end for this person. However (following, for example, Alston 1967), the terms pleasure and pain would seem to be a bit narrow to catch the wide range of experiences that seem to be relevant to a good hedonistic life. Hence, following, for example, Tännsjö (1998a), hedonism is formulated in terms of experiential well-being in this context, where something is good as an end for a person to the extent it adds to his or her experiential well-being (henceforth just well-being) and bad to the extent it lowers this well-being. In other words, it is only how a life is experienced from 'the inside' that counts when deciding whether something is good or bad for someone. However, it is of course important to notice that ill-being or a lowering of well-being at a certain time might be instrumentally valuable in bringing about greater well-being in the future. For example, it is sometimes instrumentally good for us to undergo surgery and accept the lowering of well-being associated with surgery if we thereby avoid greater lowering of well-being or achieve greater well-being in the future.[2]

Desire fulfilment theory

Desire fulfilment theory can be formulated in different ways but in a rather simplified form it can be said to claim that the more of a person's actual (intrinsic)[3] desires he or she gets fulfilled, the better it is for him or her. It is implied that these desires can be both negative and positive, i.e. they also include aversions to things or situations. In its unrestricted form the fulfilment of any actual intrinsic desires will add to the value of the person's life. It is also the case that the stronger a desire is the more valuable it will be to have it fulfilled, and in a way similar to hedonistic theory, how well off a person is at a certain moment will be a function of the amount of desire fulfilment at that moment (Brülde 1998).

This implies that if I desire something and this desire is fulfilled it will be good for me whether it positively affects my well-being or not and regardless of what I desire. For example, if I desire to be humiliated (since I might believe that I deserve it or for whatever reason) it will be good for me to have this desire fulfilled, even if it plausibly causes me to suffer. In a sense, that might be one of the important features of humiliation that makes me desire it.

A possible problem with desire fulfilment, is that we can have conflicting desires that cannot be fulfilled at the same time. For example, I might desire to be both fully conscious and without pain, which might be impossible to achieve at the same time. And if these desires are equally strong it would seem indifferent to the value of that person's life whether we fulfil one or the other of these desires. Another feature of unrestricted desire fulfilment theory is that my desires might be fulfilled without me knowing about it and this would then still be good for me. So if I desire that my close ones will be able to find comfort in my dying, and they are present when I finally go into a coma, it will be good for me according to this theory.[4]

With both hedonistic theory and desire fulfilment theory we could claim that there is little chance of arriving at valid universal claims, since different people are likely to desire different things or achieve well-being from different things in dying and death. However, there might be restrictions to these theories, which will be brought into the discussion when relevant, and these restrictions might be reasons in favour of more universal claims. Moreover, in many cases desire fulfilment theory will tend to collapse into or result in the same conclusions as the hedonistic approach or the objective list approach (presented below), since people's intrinsic desires are often about things like well-being, autonomy and intimate relationships, i.e. factors found in hedonism and on the objective list.

Objective list theory

In an objective list approach there are things that are good for me whether I desire them or not and whether they positively affect my well-being or not (and even if they negatively affect it or even if I have an aversion to them). However, well-being might very well be on the objective list and compete with these other values (and it has been argued that it must be included on any plausible list: see Brülde 1998: 46).

I do not here provide a full account of what might be on such a list but just those suggestions that seem to be the most interesting and fruitful ones to discuss in relation to a good death. In the literature (see Brülde 1998 for a good review) we find a number of different factors for what makes for a good life. Before I enumerate these different possible factors it needs to be said that they might (obviously) conflict with each other. That is, we will probably not be able to realize them all in full at the same time and hence we will have difficulties balancing these conflicting factors. However, I ignore this problem in this context, mainly since all theories seem to suffer similar problems on this account.

Achievements

One idea for what adds to a person's life is that life is made better the more achievements it contains. In other words, when I engage in different activities or behave in different ways this should have certain results, the achievement of which will make my life better. Now, for an activity or behaviour to be an achievement it seems the result must have a certain value, and it must be reached by a fairly substantial effort on account of the 'achiever'; for example, in the words of James Griffin (1996: 54), 'the achievement of the kind of value that gives life a weight or point'. However, here it is important to point out that something might be an achievement for one person even if it is not for other people or objectively. That is, the achievement might be valued by the achiever even if it is not intersubjectively[5] valued or objectively valuable. That something is on the objective list does not necessarily assume that the result of the achievement must be of objective value. It might very well be claimed that what adds to your life is making achievements (according to your own standards for achievements). However, when it is said that it is important to 'make a difference' it is probably implied that the result achieved is primarily of objective or at least intersubjective value.

Intimate personal relationships

Another item on the objective list is that a life in which we are engaged in intimate personal relationships is better than a life in which we are not thus engaged. By intimate personal relationships we imply relationships between persons being characterized by things like: mutual affectionate emotions, mutual care, mutual responsibilities, joint activities and openness about emotions and thoughts (see Griffin 1986: 67–8). We might have such relations with, for example, friends, lovers and partners. Apart from defining an intimate personal relationship, these features might also vary in such a relationship, and to the extent that these factors affect the goodness of intimate personal relationships, the goodness of our lives will vary accordingly.

Reality contact

It has also been suggested that a life in which we live in contact with reality is better than a life in which we do not live in such a contact. What this means is, however, far from clear.

In an obvious sense we are all in contact with reality since we are, first, a part of reality and, second, both influenced by and influencing on reality, so this idea must imply something beyond that. It would seem that the relevant aspects here are that I have true beliefs about reality, that I do not imagine reality to be otherwise than it is, that I do not try to avoid or deny that reality is the way it is and that my emotions are appropriate to the situation (Brülde 1998: 295). In Griffin's (1986: 67) words: 'Simply knowing about oneself and one's world is part of a good life. We value, not as instrument but for itself, being in touch with reality, being free from muddle, ignorance and mistake.' For example, if I am stopped on the street and threatened with a magnum revolver but do not get scared it might be questioned whether I am in contact with reality or if I simply imagine it to be a hoax or something along those lines. In other words, if someone threatens me with a gun it is natural or proper to become scared (given I am not a trained soldier or policeman used to facing situations like this). If I am not, it might be questioned whether I actually realize what is going on.

Being a certain kind of person

Yet another idea for what has value to people is the idea (found in, for example, Aristotle's *Nicomachean Ethics*) that a life is better in which we are certain kinds of persons or in which we exercise certain virtues. To be a certain kind of person seems to imply that we have certain character traits or dispositions that result in the way we act, behave, think, feel, react and respond. Here we can find numerous examples of such derivable ways of being or acting. For example, it is better if we act bravely and generously rather than being cowardly and mean (not primarily for the effect this might have on others but because it is good for us to be thus – which might be based on things like our true function or true nature).

Self-determination

One of the most important values in the Western context would seem to be self-determination (or autonomy, see Sandman 2004 on this) and in the following discussion this factor on the objective list is central, especially since it has been argued that much of the present view on good death within palliative care is rooted in an individualistic perspective on persons for whom it is important to control and plan the trajectory of life (see Walter 1994; Seale 1998). In this context self-determination is treated as having value as an end.[6] However, since the discussion on autonomy and self-determination is rather muddled I will briefly say something about how self-determination is understood in this context and how it is distinguished from the next item on the list, freedom. Consider the following definition (Tännsjö 1998b: 115, my translation): 'A person is . . . autonomous to the extent she does what she decides to do (because she decides to do it) and decides to do as she does because she wants it.'

Autonomy is about who and what governs our actions, i.e. about the causal connection between my wants, decisions and actions. This will henceforth be referred to as self-determination. Following the definition I might be self-determined even under very restricted circumstance, i.e. even if I do not find the alternatives of much value or do not even have many alternatives, as long as I am allowed to make the decision between the alternatives I do have. What will restrict my self-determination is if I am forced to decide or act in a way that goes against my wants or if I am manipulated into believing that the alternatives are different from what they really are. Moreover, it is important to distinguish self-determination from actually having valuable alternatives (which is dealt with under the next heading of Freedom) and also to distinguish it from actually (in the end) getting what we want (which has been dealt with under the heading of Desire fulfilment).

Freedom

The final item on our objective list, relevant to the discussion of good death, is the idea about freedom being of final value to people. Obviously this idea is closely related to the above idea about self-determination and focuses on the number of valuable alternatives we have to decide between. This might be valuable not only since it gives us the opportunity to decide in accordance with our wants but also since there is some form of end-value in just having a number of valuable alternatives (Sen 1992: 51): 'Acting freely and being able to choose are . . . directly conducive to [the good of a person[7]], not just because more freedom makes more alternatives available.'

In effect, one might claim that self-determination is about whether the actions we do are the result of our decisions and wants or not, freedom is about which alternative actions we might actually choose between and desire fulfilment is about whether the wants we have get fulfilled or not. However, it is important to emphasize that not any old alternatives will do in relation to freedom. They have to be alternatives that are important to me or that I value or want to choose between. Hence, having a large number of detergents on the shelves of our supermarket will not enhance our freedom if we do not care much about being able to choose between different detergents.

The relevance for a good dying

It seems clear that all these ideas about what is good for us, regardless of how it affects our experiential well-being or how it fulfils our desires, might be relevant in relation to a good dying. If achievements are finally valuable, does this imply that I should try to conclude the projects I am involved in before I die? If intimate personal relationships are valuable does this imply that I should be surrounded by the people I share such relationships with when dying? If it is valuable to be in contact with reality, does this imply that I should be fully aware of the fact that I am dying? If self-determination is valuable, does this imply that I should exercise self-control over problematic emotions that might crop up when facing death? Finally, if freedom is valuable, does that imply that we should know about our pending death?

These and other questions I try to deal with in the following discussion. In other words, when applicable, these different alleged factors on the objective list will be used in evaluating the goodness of proposed characteristics of a good dying.

Notes

1 The *Ars Moriendi* tradition refers to a (primarily) medieval tradition about how to end one's life in the way best suited to enable a passing to further existence in heaven rather than in hell, encompassing things like reviewing one's life, repenting sins done and fighting against the attacking demons (O'Connor 1942; Beaty 1970).
2 For a further discussion of all the different aspects of hedonism, problematic or not, see Brülde (1998).
3 By 'intrinsic' here is meant that the thing desired should be desired for its own sake, not as an instrument to something else.
4 For a further discussion of all the different aspects of desire fulfilment, problematic or not, see Brülde (1998).
5 By intersubjective value here is meant something that is valued by most people or commonly valued, or something along those lines.
6 This might be contrasted with the sense in which self-determination was used above, referring to some kind of side constraints or the like on action, which is what we generally seem to mean when we talk in terms of respect for autonomy or self-determination. If so, we should leave room for people to be self-determined or we should treat people as if they were self-determined, but there are no direct implications in terms of whether self-determination has final value or not (it might simply have instrumental value or be important to that person). This latter idea also implies that if someone does not want to exercise his or her self-determination that does not imply a value-loss to that person.
7 In the quotation from Sen it says 'well-being', but since I have given well-being a more restricted meaning, I have replaced this with the more general 'the good of the person'.

2 Dying, death and beyond

When discussing a good death it is important to be clear about what 'death' refers to. As has been touched upon before, it normally refers to the following situations: the situation in which a person *is dying* and the situation in which the person *is dead* (which lasts to the end of time according to the non-religious approach of this book). However, in between these two consecutive situations, we find a third focus of attention, namely the very event of death, i.e. the event making up the threshold between the situation of dying and the (endless) situation when the person in question is dead. The importance of distinguishing between these three aspects of our mundane notion of death has been noted by, for example, Momeyer (1988).

In the following, I refer to these three different aspects as *the period of dying, the event of death* and *post-death*, when I want to distinguish them from one another and this is not made clear by the context at hand. However, the focus of my discussion is on the period of dying and what will make this period in a person's life as good as possible – especially in relation to palliative care. The event of death is discussed only in so far as it has any bearing on the period of dying and the same applies to post-death.

There are further conceptual issues to deal with in order to clarify the general focus of this book, i.e. the period of dying. First, how should we demarcate the period of dying from the rest of life? This concerns both when the period starts and when it ends; that is, when the event of death takes place. Second, what is implied regarding the relevance of the post-death period to a person dying? Even if this period is not dealt with *per se* it might have important implications for the value of the period of dying.

Dying

Distinguishing between dying and not dying can be done in a number of different ways depending somewhat on what we need the concept of dying for. Often, attempts to define dying, or to distinguish it from death as well as from the rest of life, have been formulated in terms of a process or causal chain leading up to and causing (in its last instance) death (see, for example, Feldman 1992). For medical purposes it is of course relevant to want to know whether a certain factor is part of such a causal chain and if some form of intervention can break the chain.

This seems to be rather unproblematic, but we might complicate matters by asking whether any causal chain would do here. That is, can external processes that will lead to my death be said to imply that I am dying (for example, that a car is approaching me when I cross the road and will eventually hit me and kill me), or is it only internal processes of some sort that should be taken into consideration? An illustration of this latter problem is whether life itself is such a process (remember the joke about life being a sexually transmitted, heredity and fatal disease for which there is neither cure nor treatment[1]), and it seems difficult to formulate a clear-cut definition that would exclude life but still include what we normally take to be processes that lead to death and hence cause us to be dying. It is certainly something intuitively strange and it would provide a rather bleak picture with a definition that would cause us to be dying from the day we are born (or even from the day of conception).

This issue of vagueness in the concept of dying is of minor importance when we are discussing what makes for a good dying – especially within palliative care. The ambition of this book is not to provide criteria for when someone should receive palliative care or not (which of course is an essential question in relation to the practice of palliative care). The ambition is instead to discuss what is good when we are dying, in the sense that there is little time left in life. Thus, regardless of when and how dying starts, I will be focusing on that part of dying when we are close in time to death. Moreover, if the person has been considered a candidate for palliative care, he or she has obviously been considered to fulfil such a criterion.

This use of 'dying' implies that we might not know that we are dying. Is that a weakness in the use of the concept in relation to a good death? No, it simply means that this inclusive concept might also cover cases when it will be impossible intentionally to achieve a good dying, given, for example, that we need to change our behaviour or attitudes in the vicinity of death in order to achieve such a dying. This, however, does not wholly proclude us from taking precautions in our lives pertaining to this possibility. That is, because we can die a very sudden and unexpected death and hence our dying will be unnoticeable to us, it may be rational to organize life so that a good death or dying is achieveable even in such a case.[2] On the other hand, if a good death would need us to be aware of the fact that we are dying we should try to find criteria for assessing when death is closing in on us.

Such criteria will be along the following lines. I suffer from a disease that there is little or no hope of being cured from. I have been sentenced to death with little or no hope of being pardoned. That is, they are criteria that often will refer to the above mentioned processes or causal chains that (if I am willing to draw the conclusion) will lead me to expect to die within a short period of time. However, in this case we need to be concerned not with exactly when these processes begin, but with when we have good reasons to expect them to lead irreversibly to death, provided, of course, that we then have enough time to achieve a good dying and death.

Post-death

Before dealing with a more precise characterization of the event of death and thus of the passing from life to death, we might wonder what is implied when talking about post-death in this context. Or, simply, what is meant when we say that a person is dead in this context? What view we take on this might affect the characteristics of a good death. That is, it might affect what is good in the period of dying and it might also affect what a good event of death is.

Let me here make a distinction between two different views on what death is and call them the *religious view* and the *cessation view* respectively. All the different views that could be labelled religious have the following in common. They claim that death is not the absolute or total end of existence but a transformation into another form of existence or life. This means that, according to these views, the most important aspect of the human being (i.e. the soul, the person or whatever it is that is considered to be important) continues to exist in some form after death. Here we have a number of different alternatives: the soul or person continues to exist without being related to a body of any sort, the soul or person continues to exist together with a new or resurrected body, the soul is transformed and continues to exist in some other life-form (for example, as another person or animal or whatever). If we take a religious view on death then which religious view on death we take will of course be highly relevant to what will characterize a good death. The importance of the view we take for the period of dying and the event of death can be illustrated by the following two examples.

If we can affect what will happen to us after the event of death has taken place, the period of dying might be our last opportunity to do anything about that and hence it will be important to use that period of time wisely. This is, in effect, much of the *raison d'être* of the medieval *Ars Moriendi* tradition (Beaty 1970). Another example, taken from the Indian traditions, is the importance of the state of mind at the event of death (Firth 1993).

According to some of these traditions, the state of mind at the event of death will affect where you end up in the transmigration process. Here it makes a great difference when the event of death takes place and how the last part of the period of dying is handled.

However, since there are a number of different views that will yield different results concerning the characteristics of a good death, I will only deal with them in passing and mainly view death as if the cessation view is the correct one. This is not because I am convinced that it is the correct one but because the religious views demand that we accept a 'thick' religious description of the world and it is difficult to argue for why we should accept one such thick description before another, even if this is what we do – on faith. Moreover, for those who have a deep and serious religious faith involving ideas of an afterlife this will, to a considerable extent, show on any account of good used in this context. That is, such a person's views on dying and death are likely to be a central and important part of his or her identity and life-plan and this will of course come into play in all of the three different value approaches, since they all give ample room for the individual perspective of the person.

The event of death

Going from our main question about what characterizes a good dying and accepting the limitation of not dealing with what will happen post-death, it would still seem that we need to say something about when a person dies. In this context it will be assumed that a (human) person is an entity with at least two necessary features – a living human physical body and consciousness. If either of these is lacking – that is, if the physical body is dead or if the living physical body (irreversibly) lacks consciousness – the person will be dead. Given the cessation view as to what post-death implies, that a person is dead will, in this context, mean the same as the person not existing. On the other hand, given a religious view it would seem that the important aspect of the person continues to exist somewhere else. From any view when the person is dead the person is not coexistent with the physical body. To the extent that there is such a body it is a remaining aspect or part of the former person, hence the talk about 'remains'. Now, since it seems obvious that there can be no consciousness in a dead physical body but that there can be a living physical body without consciousness, it can be taken that the important criterion of a person's death is the physical body's irreversible loss of consciousness.

Another aspect of the event of death is that when the loss of consciousness is concurrent with the death of the physical body, as compared with when consciousness is lost without the physical body being fully dead, we will have a very differently featured event of death. In relation to this, different characteristics of good death might be applicable or relevant. Moreover, it might make a difference to the goodness of the lives of people in the vicinity of the dying person. One radical difference between these two kinds of events is that in the former case it is clearly observable when the person dies and is dead, but in the latter case this is not as obvious and calls for a careful physical examination. Furthermore, it might not be clear exactly when the event of death has taken place in the latter case. The examination will show (given the criteria) whether the physical body is post-death or not, but not exactly when this took place. In the latter case it might look as if the person is still alive, since he retains some of his bodily functions, something which, of course, might be distressing to the close ones of the (now dead) person. Another difference is that in the latter case we can remove vital internal organs for transplant without killing the person, which is not possible in the former case. This will, of course, also affect what state the physical remains will be in at the time of burial or cremation and also when this can take place. Once again, this might have repercussions on the lives of the close ones, but also on the life of the recipient of such an organ.

However, in many cases death will occur according to the 'traditional' model where the physical body stops functioning concurrently with the irreversible loss of consciousness (or rather that the latter occurs as a result of the former).

The above discussion obviously concerns the event of physical or bio-logical death, and in the discussion of good dying and death the concept of social death has been frequently referred to as yet another important event in the dying person's life (see, for example, Sudnow 1967; Walter 1994; Seale 1998; Lawton 2000). Social death refers to something like the point in time when the dying person has lost his or her important relationships and is no longer treated as a person, part of the social fabric he or she used to be a part of. It has been argued that the hospice movement, on which much of modern palliative care rests, has been a reaction to the separation of social and physical death, trying to bring them closer together. It seems to share this ambition with those who raise calls for euthanasia, even though the latter doubt the ability of palliative carers to postpone social death until it coincides with a physical death not induced by intentional activity (Seale 1998). The concept of social death does to some extent come into play in the following discussion, since on the objective list and in most people's ideas of what brings well-being and what they desire, relationships fill an important role.

The value of the event of death[3]

When dealing with the question of good dying we need to say something about the value of the event of physical death. The focus is on whether it is good or bad for a specific person to die under specific circumstances. To contrast, another interpretation could be whether it is good for persons to be mortal. These are obviously different questions, since we might claim that it is good that we are mortal but still bad that I die now (due to the circumstances), or even that it is bad that we are mortal but still good (or the best possible alternative) that I die now (due to the circumstances).

The reason for dealing with these issues is that the answer to them will, in different ways, affect what is characteristic of a good dying. Above all, it will be important in relation to when it is a good time to die, if ever. If the event of death were neither good nor bad for us it would seem to make no difference to the value of our lives when we died, at least as long as this did not influence the way in which we died, i.e. our dying. It is also relevant, since it might, for example, affect which attitude to adopt towards death in order to die a good death.

This question has to be distinguished from, but is at the same time probably related to, the question of whether what happens post-death can be good or bad for a specific person or generally for us as people. This question will not be dealt with in this context. If what happens when we are dead can affect the value of our lives we need to take that into account when evaluating how the event of death will affect the value of life.

In the following I draw mainly on the discussion by Frances Kamm (1993) in her *Morality, Mortality*, where she discusses several different factors for why death might be bad or good for us. Here I focus on the deprivation factor (the D-factor for short) and the extinction factor (the E-factor). Another argument that is briefly discussed is that found in Dworkin (1993), according to which death is bad to the extent that it wastes the investment that is made into that life. In line with the above we could call this the waste factor (or W-factor for short). Let us start with the D-factor, which Kamm thinks is the most important reason for why death is bad for us.

The deprivation factor

The deprivation factor says something along the following lines. Death is bad for us when it deprives us of future 'goods' or a future good life, while it is good for us when it deprives us of a future bad life. In other words, loss of future 'goods' or 'bads' does not necessarily matter for a bad or good death, but the loss of a future good/bad *life* does. That is, since death might deprive us of both a close relationship (which is presumably something good) and an abundance of suffering (which is presumably something bad) we need to look at the overall value of the stretch of life we are deprived of in death.

To the extent that death is bad it is described as something comparatively bad in terms of our death being compared to a situation in which we would have remained alive and the life that we would have continued to live. If this latter life would have been a good life, we can conclude that death was indeed bad for us. So the D-factor could be formulated in the following way:

- If death deprives me of a future good life, then death is bad for me.
- If death deprives me of a future bad life, then death is good for me.[4]
- If death deprives me of a future indifferent or neutral life, then death is indifferent for me.

Exactly what death deprives me of would seem to depend on what perspective we assume. For example, we might ask whether it is good or bad that the person dies at a specific time T or we might ask whether it is good or bad that the person dies *per se*. Furthermore, it is not unreasonable to claim that it was good for someone to die at T given the disease she was suffering from but still claim that, on the whole, it was bad for her to die. That is, the combination of suffering from the disease and dying was bad for her, even if once having suffered the disease the best alternative might have been to die (see Momeyer 1988: 20–1).

On the whole, it seems as if death is, at best, the least bad option given the circumstances we face and it would have been better for us had we not faced these circumstances. That is, death is never or almost never actually good for us, on the whole (see Sandman 2001).

The extinction factor

Before turning to Dworkin's argument about waste we will take a look at Kamm's other factor, the extinction factor. This idea implies death to be bad owing to its depriving me of all possibilities of anything significant happening in the future. According to Kamm this feature of death is distinguishable from the D-factor in that here one is concerned more with life and its prospects 'being all over' than with the goods of a possible future life that one has been deprived of (see also Furley 1986). However, it is not very clear exactly what the E-factor might amount to, and two different interpretations come to mind. The first is the idea that life in itself has value, apart from any other features it might have, what is normally called *vitalism*. Since this idea does not seem plausible to me because it implies that even a life full of the worst of suffering would still be worth living if it continued for long enough, I focus on the latter idea in this context.

The other interpretation of the E-factor is that the length of life matters, that it is important that *I* will be around for as long as possible. This is, presumably, a better interpretation of what Kamm means when she talks about the E-factor. Compare two lives, containing an equal balance of 'goods' and 'bads', but of unequal length. According to this interpretation of the E-factor, even if we do not make a value gain, it is better to be around for longer. Hence, not only further good life might be a reason to postpone

death but also a further amount of neutral life. Since it would seem important to me that *I* am still alive for some time I seem to have reasons for going
on with life for some time if it does not make a difference to the value of my
life, i.e. if future life is neutral to me (see Sandman 2001). Kamm actually
claims that people who are dying might want a few extra days – even if these
will not contain any significant goods – as a buffer zone before death.

What about continuation of a bad life? Since it is not implied that length
of life has final value it seems more doubtful whether extra length should be
bought at the cost of a bad life. In this context, it will be assumed that a
longer life is not worth the price of a bad life. Assuming that length of life
has final value would imply that even the most torturous suffering might be
made up for with a long enough life of neutral value or even of slightly
negative value (depending on how we value length) – something that is
intuitively unconvincing.

In conclusion, I find that even if the E-factor does not change whether
death is good or bad for us in the case of future life being neutral, it will give
us a reason to continue our lives until death becomes good for us (or any
future life is bad for us). The reason for this is that it seems to make a
difference whether I am around in the world for a shorter or longer period.

The waste factor

Finally, we will take a look at a suggestion by Dworkin (1993), according to
which death is bad to the extent that it wastes our investments[5] in our own
lives. Dworkin claims that any existing human life involves a number of
investments that would yield no benefits if this life were to end (pre-
maturely). These investments are of two different kinds: investments on
behalf of nature or God (whatever we prefer), and investments on behalf of
the person living the life, his or her parents, other people and the culture.

We can follow Dworkin's line of reasoning, which starts with the need to
explain the different attitudes we generally have towards the death of a
young person versus the death of an old person:

> the frustration [prompted by a person's death] is greater if it
> takes place after rather than before the person has made a significant
> personal investment in his own life, and less if it occurs after any
> investment has been substantially fulfilled, or as substantially fulfilled
> as is anyway likely.
>
> (Dworkin 1993: 88)

According to this, he considers it worse to die when you are young enough
to have made investments but not old enough to have seen them fulfilled. But
if you are younger or older than that, it is less bad. However, it seems a bit
strange to discuss this in terms of age, since we might have made substantial

investments at an early age or less substantial investments even at a fairly high age. Hence, in the following I simply assume that the actual investment made in a life is the relevant criterion for whether death is good or bad, regardless of at what age the person dies.

As Dworkin observes, death is not the only way in which our investment can be frustrated: 'it can be frustrated by other forms of failure: by handicaps or poverty or misconceived projects or irredeemable mistakes or lack of training or even brute bad luck' (*ibid.*: 89). For this reason he seems to consider it an open question whether death is always the worst frustration conceivable or if we have to evaluate each specific case and see which is the worst cause of frustration in that case. Conversely, we may also imagine more peculiar investments such that death is their yield – in which case death is good for these persons. For example, Christ dedicated his life to follow his father's will and save the world. As it happens (or rather, as is believed), his death was the fulfilment of that investment and hence *ceteris paribus* good for him according to the W-factor.

All in all, then, death is always bad to the extent that it frustrates the investments of life, although not necessarily the worst that can happen in this vein. Death is good to the extent that it fulfils or is the fruit of our investments. In the cases where no investments are frustrated (either because none have been made or because the person has already benefited from the yields of the investments made) it would seem that death is not bad or good but indifferent to the person dying. However, for the normal person, there will always remain *some* yield to collect from made investments, so death will always be bad to that extent.[6]

Dworkin distinguishes the waste idea from the deprivation idea in that it is grounded in facts about the life already lived, which the D-factor is not. However, true as this may seem, it is still the case that the W-factor can, at least partly, be described in terms of us being deprived of the fulfilment of investments made and hence the W-factor seems to be a sub-category of the D-factor. There seems to be a significant difference though, relating not to the deprivation of yields but to the waste associated with the investments. When we make an investment that is supposed to yield some benefit in the future we generally forsake some good now for the sake of some greater good in the future, and we might even have to suffer something bad for the sake of this future good. For example, I have in trying to make a career for myself in philosophy forsaken other (well paid, secure) careers or jobs as well as a number of enjoyments, desires and achievements I have had or could have had. If death cuts me short of pursuing such a career I am not only deprived of that career but I have also wasted the investments made to be able to pursue such a career (not altogether, since I have enjoyed doing it on occasion). Hence, the W-factor also seems to claim something about the life we have lived until death and how that directly affects the value of death (see Sandman 2001).

What the discussion shows is that the W-factor goes beyond the D-factor and might even, occasionally, turn the balance of the value of death. Situations where the W-factor can turn the balance and does not merely emphasize the D-factor seem quite rare and hence the W-factor plays only a minor role in the following discussion.

Summary

Let us summarize the conclusions we have reached in relation to the different factors discussed, i.e. the deprivation factor, the extinction factor and the waste factor.

We have found that the most important factor in making death good or bad is the deprivation factor, which implies that death is bad for us to the extent that it deprives us of future good life and good for us to the extent that it deprives us of future bad life. The D-factor should be supplemented by the W-factor, which brings in the cost of investments made when we have not yet benefited from the yield of these investments. This will often emphasize the badness of death implied by the D-factor but will, on occasion, turn the balance in relation to the D-factor, making death bad when the D-factor implies it to be neutral or slightly good.

The E-factor turns out not to make a difference to the goodness or badness of death but gives us a reason to go on with life also when future life is neutral, until the point where future life becomes bad for us (and, hence, death good).

In this chapter it has been argued that death is generally something bad for us and when it is good for us, this is due to us being in a situation that it would have been better not to be in. In other words, when death is good, it is actually the least bad of the options at hand. This conclusion plays an important role in the following when we discuss what makes for a good dying. If death is indeed bad for us, this should presumably show in the way we relate to death – especially if we do not have a purely hedonistic theory of value. We do generally consider it rational to fear what is bad for us, or to protest and fight against what is bad for us, or to try to avoid it in different ways. Hence, in the following the general badness of death is the contrasting background against which the different suggestions for what makes for a better dying and death will have to be judged.

Conclusions and relevance to palliative care

In this chapter we have discussed how to interpret talk about good death and it was argued that we might distinguish between the period of dying, the event of death and post-death. Dying is characterized by the fact that it is the last period of life just before we die, regardless of whether there is an internal or external process that has started and will lead to our death. Given such a view on dying, it will not always be possible to tell whether someone is dying or not. For palliative care it is of course important to know whether someone is dying or not, since that is one of the criteria for whether the person in question should receive palliative care or not. Still, those who are receiving palliative care have been judged to be close to death, and hence the discussion of what we should do when dying is at least relevant to people within palliative care.

It has been argued that the event of biological death is characterized by the person irreversibly lacking consciousness, which of course implies that a person's death is not always clearly observable from the outside (i.e when the person is brain-dead but the physical body still lingers on). This is obviously relevant to palliative care, since within palliative care there are also ideas on how to deal with dead persons and how to care for close ones when the patient is dead. Moreover, when the event of biological death takes place is also relevant, since it has been argued that the palliative movement (or more specifically the hospice movement) is, in part, motivated by an attempt to bring biological and social death closer together. However, when the event of death takes place has no real bearing on the discussion of this book.

What characterizes post-death for a person can obviously be relevant to palliative care in the sense that people's beliefs about post-death will probably influence their lives and what they want when in palliative care. However, I have chosen not to deal with this explicitly in this book.

In this chapter we have also dealt with the question of what value death at a certain time has to the person who dies. It has been argued that the most important factor for judging what value death has is the so-called deprivation factor, which implies that the value of death at a certain time is decided by what death will deprive me of compared to if I die later. It has also been argued that this implies that death is generally bad for us and, when it is good, this is because of our being in an overall bad situation. Hence, at best, death is the least bad of all bad alternatives. Both these conclusions, if sound, are relevant to palliative care. First, since the deprivation factor implies that there might come a time when I am better off dead, it should be discussed whether this has normative implications in terms of whether we induce death or a death-like condition at such a time. Second, the conclusion that death is generally bad for us should perhaps somewhat dampen or balance the tendencies within palliative care to become a 'happy death movement' (Lofland 1978).

Notes

1 I owe this pun to Christian Munthe.
2 Of course, this may be a source of conflict, since taking such precautions far in advance might preclude us from pursuing projects etc. that we would have done if we had viewed ourselves as immortal or with a long life ahead.
3 For a more thorough discussion of this see Sandman (2001).
4 This is even supported in the Bible, in Ecclesiastes, where we find: 'Death is better than a miserable life' (see Badham 1996 for a Christian defence of euthanasia drawing on this idea).
5 Having made investments in our own life means that we have given time and effort to projects that will not reward us until further on in our lives. For example, I have invested a lot of time and effort in this book – something that I hope will reward me when I have finished it.
6 With the extended notion of investment, and to the extent that we accept all of the mentioned alternatives as investments, there are always some frustrated investments and hence every death is bad.

3 | Global features of death and dying

This first chapter on specific ideas about good death and dying deals with whether death and dying should have what I call global features; that is, whether death and dying should have certain features in order to be good. Here I discuss whether death and dying should be consistent with the rest of life or not, whether death and dying should be meaningful or not and whether death and dying should be dignified or not. In the following chapters we move on to ideas about more specific actions and attitudes to perform and have in dying.

A consistent death

In Avery Weisman's account of an appropriate death we find the following criteria:

> Our hypothesis is that, whatever its content, an appropriate death must satisfy four principal requirements: (1) conflict is reduced; (2) compatibility with the ego ideal is achieved; (3) continuity of important relations is preserved or restored; (4) consummation of a wish is brought about.
>
> (Weisman and Hackett 1961: 248)

> Given a little choice and autonomy, what death would be best for us, the death most consistent with the values and aims we have followed throughout life?
>
> (Weisman 1974: 139)

Drawing on Weisman's formulations about the consistency of death, we find two different ways of expression, somewhat different in meaning: first, that death should be consistent with the values and aims we actually follow; second, that death should be consistent with our ego ideal. Moreover, we might look at consistency from a synchronic perspective as well as from a diachronic perspective. Consequently, we have four different interpretations of the idea about consistency to be dealt with in this context: (a) death and dying should be synchronically consistent with the values and aims we follow; (b) death and dying should be synchronically consistent with our ideal values and aims; (c) death and dying should be diachronically consistent with the values and aims we have followed throughout our lives; (d) death and dying should be diachronically consistent with the ideal values and aims we have had throughout our lives.

Since synchronic and diachronic consistency would amount to the same thing, given that we have not changed values, or ideals about values, in relation to diachronic consistency I will only look at the case when we do not have the same values or ideals about values in dying that we have had throughout the rest of our lives, or actually the values and ideals we have had throughout the greater part of our lives, since we might have changed values and ideals a number of times. This would seem to be a problem for the diachronic idea, i.e. that it is difficult to decide the relevant set of values or ideals that death and dying should be consistent with. In a sense, the whole idea about consistency seems to rest on the idea that we have well established and well defined self-identities, which should influence the way we die – something that might not be true. However, in this context I will ignore this problem and assume that we can indeed find the relevant set. This idea about being consistent with the values and ideals I have had in life would seem to match well the idea, found in, for example Walter (1994) and Seale (1998), about modern good dying being portrayed in terms of how it fits the life-project of the dying person.

Weisman (1973: 370) claims that: 'death at any age can still be compatible with everything that the person stood for during life . . . what a person *represented* in terms of an ego ideal'. An ego ideal is a set of norms and values for how *I* should act or behave or be. Being an *ideal*, it is, presumably, not something we accord with at the moment (at least not to the full), but something we strive towards and want to accord with. By an *ego* ideal is probably meant that it is the ideal *I* adhere to concerning how I should act, be and behave, which do not necessarily accord with the majority view or the official view, even if I am influenced by such views.

Synchronic consistency

First we deal with whether we have reason to die in a way that is synchronically consistent with our present values, ideal or not. Is it not logically true that we always act and behave in a way consistent with the values and aims we actually follow, i.e. it seems to be implied by the very expression 'actually follow'? If so, it would seem empty to claim that this is what it takes to die a better or good death.

A problem here is that the set of values and aims we follow is not necessarily internally consistent; or it is far from likely that it is internally consistent. Hence, whatever we do, it is likely to be inconsistent with some of the values and aims we actually follow at the same time that it is consistent with other values and aims followed by us. If so, the idea would be that we would be better off if the set of values and aims we actually follow was internally consistent. However, what you actually do would seem more important (from a value perspective) than whether your actions are internally consistent in what they express in terms of values and aims. For example, if you always act in a way that causes yourself suffering and in a way that is expressive of a degrading self-image, it would obviously be better if you did not act internally consistently and sometimes acted so as not to cause yourself suffering.

Now, even if we act in a way that is consistent with all the values we actually follow, i.e. this set is internally consistent, we might still not act in accordance with our ideal set of values and aims. On the face of it, ideal values and aims probably being more basic and important to us, we would seem to benefit by dying in accordance with them. However, the problem with internal consistency still holds – hence, we might have a basic desire to die in a way that is not consistent with other values and aims (i.e. basic desires) we have.

Consider the following example. A dying person is a fundamentalist Christian who strongly believes in the sanctity of life and is therefore an ardent opponent of euthanasia and terminal sedation. However, she is rather 'squeamish' and views pain as one of the worst things that can happen to her, so she strongly desires to die a death without pain. Her fatal disease develops in a way that ends in a situation where her excruciating pains can only be managed by terminal sedation or euthanasia. Which death is most consistent with her values, aims or desires at that point? That is, should she endure the pain or compromise her fundamentalist beliefs? From a desire fulfilment approach, if her strongest and most basic desire is to get rid of the pain then she should probably go for the sedation or even the euthanasia. Likewise, from a hedonistic approach, she should probably choose sedation or euthanasia, since that would seem to tally better with her well-being than the pain would (even taking into account the satisfaction of being consistent with her overall values and aims). On the other hand, she may have equally strong, basic and conflicting desires in this situation and it might be impossible to decide which one to fulfil. The point here is simply that in few (if any) cases are the values and aims we have in life wholly consistent with each other – hence, it might sometimes be difficult to find the death most consistent with these values and aims given the situations dying and death might leave us in. In Lawton (2000) the pressing and non-negotiable problems disease, and the bodily decay following in its wake, could face us with are extremely well described.

To continue the example above, this person might also, when actually facing the situation where euthanasia or terminal sedation would be a possible solution, realize that she cannot accept the consequences of her important values and aims (which she has accepted earlier) even if she still would like to be able to adhere to these values and aims. So, first, we are not likely always to have full insight into what is consistent with our values and aims in life and might not accept this when we realize what it is. Second, we might have accepted them theoretically, but when faced with the situations where they become real options, we realize that it is impossible for us to accept them in practice.

Now, even if we have an ego ideal that would not make for a worse death if accorded with, it is not clear what it entails for a death (and dying) to be compatible with this ideal. Consider the following example. A person has a rather stoical ego ideal and wants to endure the suffering he encounters. However, he cannot fully personify this ideal and, hence, in the face of great suffering he will become a rather pitiful and deplorable figure (according to his own standards). Which would be the death most compatible with his ideal: a death in which he faces great suffering and tries to endure but fails and, hence, compromises his ideals; or a death in which he does not face great suffering and does not compromise his ideal but, on the other hand, does not realize or express it either? That is, even if the latter situation does not compromise his ideals it is not compatible with his ego ideal in the sense of giving him an opportunity to act it out.

Moreover, with the ideal being just an *ideal*, we do not generally live up to it and, as dying is generally a situation in which our powers and abilities decline, the ideal might be even more difficult to accord with when dying (Lawton 2000). Hence, even if compatibility with the ego ideal might be important in most cases, there is something unrealistic about the idea that we should be able to die in a way compatible with our ego ideal.

Diachronic consistency

Let us move on to the idea about diachronic consistency between, on the one hand, dying and death and, on the other, the values and aims we have actually followed throughout the major part of our life, or the ego ideal we have had. In this context I focus on the situation when we have different values and aims in dying from the ones we followed or had as our ego ideal earlier in life.[1]

The first version of this idea seems to suffer the same problems as the idea about synchronic consistency, i.e. since our set of values and aims is seldom internally consistent a certain action might be consistent with some of the earlier values and aims and inconsistent with others. Hence, we might have trouble deciding whether someone is acting diachronically consistent or not.

Moreover, it is difficult to see why we should be consistent with the values and aims we used to follow, especially when these values and aims are morally problematic, or when they are problematic in relation to what is in our own best interest. Hence, diachronic consistency of the values and aims we actually follow has in itself no special support from the different value approaches and will depend on how such consistency best furthers what is valuable as ends.

A possible exception to this would be if by being inconsistent we lose out on the yield from an investment made earlier in life, i.e. what was presented as the waste factor for what makes death bad for us. If such a yield would have compensated us for the cost of the investment, it seems our lives are made somewhat worse for including a cost with no corresponding benefit. However, once again, this is only relevant when we would actually benefit from the yield of the investment and there is such a cost associated with that investment. This is a cost in terms of time or effort or whatever that we presumably chose to pay in the belief that we would be diachronically consistent. Furthermore, if this yield is replaced by something that adds even more value to our life, it seems we have not lost anything from an overall perspective.

Finally, we should deal with the question of whether we would die a better death to the extent that such a death is diachronically consistent with the ideal values and aims we have had throughout our lives. It was accepted above that to die in accordance with one's ideal values and aims has fairly strong support, even if the characteristics of dying might not enable us to do so. Could we draw a similar conclusion when it comes to diachronic consistency?

Returning again to our ardent opponent of euthanasia and terminal sedation in the example above, she stuck to her values and aims but allowed herself to be inconsistent or accepted a failure in relation to these. Now we imagine that she reconsiders her former ideas and comes to hold a different and opposing set of values and aims concerning euthanasia and terminal sedation. Hence, a death in which she receives terminal sedation would be consistent with her present values and aims, but not with the values and aims held throughout the greater part of her life.

Would she die a worse death for having been sedated if this is not diachronically consistent with the rest of her life? There might be some different suggestions as to why it would be bad for her. One is that her present values and aims are adopted under duress, or less than optimal conditions, and the values and aims held through the greater part of her life are more in line with what she would have wanted had she been fully rational or in more optimal circumstances.[2] Another is that in dying a death not consistent with the values and aims of the greater part of her life, she would seem to have lived her life in vain and made it of lesser value than it would have been had she died in a way consistent with that life.

If we first consider the idea about the present values being adopted under duress, it might be argued that the values and aims we have should, to be as rational and well founded as possible, be adopted in full knowledge of the situations they concern. For example, to be able to assess whether it is good to be adopted or not, we should try to picture the situation of having been adopted as vividly as possible, in all its different aspects (if not actually having this experience), so that we are then able to pass a well considered judgement about the value of adoption to the adopted child. If this is a plausible view of how we should arrive at our important values and aims in life then values and aims concerning situations of duress might even benefit from experiencing such situations, since we might not be able to picture them as vividly as needed otherwise. However, for these values and aims to be well considered, they should not be arrived at or changed lightly and, following this, if experiencing dying makes us re-evaluate our formerly held values and aims we should probably give some time and thought before we accept a more definitive change resulting in accepting previously non-accepted ways to die. Still, having earlier held strong and well considered views on good dying and death might imply taking even more seriously any change in these views – taking them to account for a fundamental change, not just a change by whim (if, indeed, we find it important that our values and aims should be well considered).

Here is a real example.[3] A woman, formerly a nurse and author of books on palliative care (and presumably, given the general attitudes of palliative care personnel, a former opponent of euthanasia), approached her physician to receive permanent relief from her distressing symptoms (implying that she wanted to receive euthanasia). Since this took place in Sweden, where euthanasia is legally prohibited, the physician could not grant her wish and instead found it best to approach her further in conversation to find out what her wish amounted to. However, the important question here is whether to interpret her wish as a sincere reconsideration of her previous values and aims or not. Since she spent her life working with and thinking about palliative care I find it plausible that we should interpret her wish not as uttered lightly but as a well considered change of values and aims; to some extent for the very reason that it contradicts her earlier values and aims in life. That is, I think it is likely that we generally want to be consistent with the values and aims we hold through life and we might find it costly to change our views; especially for the reason that the values and aims we have are generally an important part of our identity, and we might view a funda-mental change of values as a fundamental change of who we are. Hence, when someone has changed her mind about something of fundamental importance to her this should at face value be taken to imply that her 'new' views are well considered and serious.

From the perspective of self-determination we should take seriously the desires held at the particular point in question without looking at earlier or later desires, and allow people to arrange their lives in accordance with those present desires to the extent that this is morally acceptable.

What about the other suggestion that, in changing the overall values and aims of our lives when approaching death, we will make the greater part of our life of lesser value to us or waste that life or make those earlier values and aims seem to be held in vain.[4] First, to the person we were when we held those views and lived accordingly, they would seem to be of value and hence not wasted. That is, the problem occurs if we, as we normally do, view these different points in time as parts of the same person's life, and not as parts of different, but consecutive, persons. Let us assume this straighforward view on persons here. Would this argument be potent in such a case?

As was argued in relation to the W-factor, if our values and aims have made us forsake things in the past in order to benefit in the future and we, in giving up these values and aims, do not get the expected benefits we will to some extent have wasted our lives, presupposing that the expected benefits really were benefits and we really did forsake something to get these benefits. Hence, if we have worked for the greater part of our life, forsaking family and pleasures, to solve a scientific problem and when closing in on it just give the project up, then we will obviously have wasted a large amount of time and effort that could have been better spent. However, it is not consistency *per se* that is important here, but whether we have forsaken anything of value in the past and whether the yield would be of value to us. If we have not forsaken anything we will not lose out because of inconsistency (if the loss of the yield is outweiged by some other gain) or alternatively if we have forsaken something in the past this is not made better if consistency results in us getting something that is not of value to us.

Moreover, that it is better not to change one's ideal values has nothing to do with the former life getting wasted or with consistency, since we have already benefited from that life and cannot be deprived of these benefits. It is only relevant if the change results in a worse life. Hence, once again, diachronic consistency is important when it implies continuing a good life and prevents a change for the worse, but not if it prevents a change for the better.

Summary

Following the above discussion, we can conclude that the idea that death and dying should be synchronically consistent with the ideal values and aims we have at the time of dying has fairly strong support. A problem in relation to the idea about consistency is that our values and aims are normally not internally consistent, something that will result in difficulties in judging what is the dying and death most consistent with these values and aims.

We found support for the idea about diachronic consistency if we assumed that we had made an investment earlier in life and we would lose out on the yield that investment would have brought us if we did not lead diachronically consistent lives. However, this depends on whether the investment implies a cost to us or not, and also whether the yield of the investment will be compensated by something else or not. Hence, it would seem that this idea would only be relevant in a small number of cases. It was also given support if changing our values, ideal or not, would imply that we added less value to our lives, meaning that a change for the better is of course good for us, despite it being diachronically inconsistent.

Moreover, we found a positive reason for changing our mind in dying to the extent that we want our values and aims to be well considered. That is, if we want our values and aims to take into account the true nature of the situation and experiencing the situation will make us change them, it might be taken as evidence that they are indeed well considered after such a change.

Normative aspects of a consistent death

As the discussion shows, it is an open question whether a consistent dying and death will bring about a good life for the patient and close ones at the end of life. Hence, a consistent death cannot be a goal of care for every individual patient or close one.

In line with this, the best normative strategy of the professional carer is to let the patient decide on the best way to die, without looking at in which way this is consistent with the patient's former or present values and aims; unless the patient is adamant about wanting to die in a way that is consistent with a certain set of values and aims. In such a case, the carer should obviously help the patient to fashion a dying that is consistent. Here it is obvious that the patient and the close ones might have different views as to whether death and dying should be consistent or not. However, to the extent that adapting to patients' wants does not seriously hurt the close ones, carers have reasons to prioritize how the patients want their death and dying to be fashioned.

When helping the patient and the close ones to such a death, carers need to ensure that the care fulfils the demands of justice. That is, patients should not be helped to a consistent death at the expense of other patients.

Neither is the carer obligated to provide care or treatment that is not proven to be effective. To the extent that there is no definite risk involved, they could provide care with no such proven effectiveness. However, this could not be done at the expense of justice, i.e. carers are not obliged to provide care or treatment or in other ways to help patients in ways that will be unfair to other dying patients and close ones in their care.

When carers are helping the patient and his or her close ones to a consistent death, they cannot be obliged to risk their own good life. This is, to some extent, dependent on things like whether carers have access to counselling and whether they are well prepared to handle these kinds of situations, which in turn will depend on things like their degree of education and experience. To exemplify, if it is in line with the dying person's values to treat other people as of lesser worth, carers do not have to accept this.

Since a consistent death does not have reasons to support a universal application, it is essential that palliative care philosophy does not contain any preconceived views on whether it is better to die a consistent death or not. Instead, as indicated above, carers should have an open mind as to what dying and death the patient and his or her close ones want.

A meaningful death

We now turn to the idea that it is important to find meaning in death in order to get a good death. Callahan (1993: 195) states: 'I want to find meaning in my death or, if not a full meaning, a way of reconciling myself to it. Some kind of sense must be made of my mortality.'[5] First, we will explore what it implies to say that a death has meaning. Second, we will take a look at some different suggestions for what exactly makes death meaningful found in Callahan (1993), Elias (1985) and Singer (1996).

Frankl (1963) says that suffering is suffering only when it is bereft of meaning, and Callahan (1993: 95–6) claims that: 'the meaning attributed to the pain will make a great difference in how oppressive the pain is taken to be'. From this I think that we can interpret 'meaning' to imply that the pain or suffering has some purpose to it, i.e. that it is instrumental in relation to some goal (which is valuable) and hence has instrumental value. But there might be more to this idea about meaning:

> In using the term 'meaning', I want to encompass three elements: our way of understanding and explaining our human situation; the value we attach to our lives; the sense of emotional wholeness and integrity we experience, the way in which the cognitive and valuative blend together.
>
> (Callahan 1993: 166)

Following this, if we can understand and explain our dying and death, if this understanding results in us attaching value to dying and death and if these two aspects, together with the emotions we experience in relation to dying and death, are coherent or integrated, then, it seems, we have found meaning in the situation, something that would then make for a better death.

Meaning as making for a good death?

Beginning with the first part about understanding and explaining, I will take it that these are different sides of a similar coin, where explaining implies communicating understanding of a situation. Henceforth, I will only talk in terms of understanding.

To understand dying and death would seem to imply that we are able to find reasonable answers to questions like: Why do we die at all? Why do I die the way I do? Do we have to die? Is it good that we die? However, even if the understanding involves answers that describe the physiological processes that will cause us to die, in general or individually, it is not mainly such an understanding that seems to be called for in the search for meaning, especially if one is not satisfied with the answers provided by medicine or science, one of the reasons why the hospice and palliative movement sees itself as an alternative to traditional medicine in relation to death and dying (Seale 1998).

What we need to find when inquiring into the meaning of dying and death is an answer to the question of what purpose my death or dying fulfils or simply what value it has to me; and it would not seem totally satisfactory if the answer provided is that it has no value or purpose. Callahan (1993: 224) admits that finding meaning in this sense might be problematic: 'My death . . . can make sense even if I find that sense intolerable. At least I can understand what is happening. It is even better, to be sure, if I can find some justification for the way things are, but that may not be possible.' At the same time, the quotation indicates that understanding the situation of dying and death is better than not being able to make any sense at all of it, something that the hedonistic theory does not generally seem to agree upon. That is, from a hedonistic standpoint it is sometimes better to live with the unfounded idea that death and dying has a certain purpose or value, even when in fact it has not. On the other hand, from a desire fulfilment perspective, our desires will not be fulfilled until death and dying really has purpose or value.

If Callahan is right and understanding the situation should always make us better off, we need to resort to the objective list approach. In this approach we find the idea that a true understanding of the situation (or being in contact with reality, which would seem to amount to something similar) has final value.

However, we might accept a hostility-restriction on this idea, implying that when the situation or reality is hostile to us, and dying and death are candidates for such situations, understanding it or being in contact with it would not make us better off. Are we, for example, really better off knowing everything people think about us, especially when people do not like us? Hence, whether a true understanding of the situation will make for a better death depends on which version of the reality contact idea we accept. A problem for Callahan here is that he does not seem to subscribe to the view that we should have a true understanding of the situation, since he repeatedly emphasizes the need to *create* meaning or *give* dying and death meaning:

> The *meaning we will attach* to pain and suffering is shaped over the course of our lives. Our history, our culture, our personal structure of understanding will all make a difference to this meaning, but they will be blended in different ways in different people ... They did not choose to suffer, and they did not deserve to suffer, but they took that circumstance and *created meaning* ... Death can be *given a meaning*, though imperfectly, if we find a way to understand it as a 'part of life'.
>
> (Callahan 1993: 132, 151, 167, emphasis added)

If this is a correct interpretation of Callahan, meaning does not imply a *true* understanding of dying and death and will not be supported by the idea about reality contact. Instead, these claims indicate that Callahan might be after the hedonistic benefits of meaning, if anything.

As indicated above, it is not enough that we understand why death and dying happen to us; we should also find that our death and dying have some value or purpose. Generally when we talk about the meaning of life, we might mean either that life has a certain value or quality, i.e that life contains well-being, or that we have control over our lives or some other values (Seale 1998). However, we might also mean that life fulfils some purpose, i.e. has instrumental value to something or someone outside ourselves. Perhaps this latter interpretation best catches what we generally mean, and we might be instrumentally valuable to other people or in relation to some higher purpose or in some other sense. Once again, this is supported in all the value approaches, i.e. if we find it important to be instrumentally valuable, we will find well-being in being so and we will thereby fulfil an important desire; on the objective list we are likely to find support in such a view given, for example, the idea about relationships (Walter 1994).

Walter (1994) argues (in line with others) that most people nowadays have to fashion meaning for themselves on their own and the ready-made meaning stories about the purpose of human life and of my life are lost. Hence, I have to find out what purpose my life and my death will have and might not be able to fall back on the ideas of meaning given by the world religions or world philosophies. Or, at least, I will have to try to pick and choose among these religions and philosophies.

Callahan argues that apart from the two conditions above being satisfied, there should be no conflict between our understanding of the situation, our evaluation of the situation and the emotions we have in relation to the situation. This is elaborated in the following way: 'Unless we can blend our thinking, and feeling and wanting into some integrated whole, we will find ourselves torn apart – our reason fighting our values – with nothing adding up in our interior lives' (Callahan 1993: 166). Perhaps it is a bit odd to claim that the last part is needed to find meaning in a situation (as we normally use the concept of meaning), but at least from a hedonistic perspective it might be needed to make meaningfulness good for us. If knowing that we have fulfilled a certain purpose will not bring comfort or satisfaction to us, we will not benefit (hedonistically) from such knowledge. This is less important from the other value perspectives, since in them it is enough that we actually have fulfilled such a purpose, even if we have difficulties taking comfort in it given the price we have to pay, i.e. dying and death.

We might ask whether it is reasonable that we actually find such a meaning in our dying and death, however good it would be, and in the following we take a look at some ideas about why death and dying would have meaning.

Callahan's meaning

Callahan claims that meaningful death draws on two essential elements of understanding:

> One of them is an understanding of death as an event that is ever foreshadowed during life, a life made up of 'little deaths'. The other is an understanding that life and death are inextricably intertwined and that much of the value of death comes because of this relationship, not despite it.
>
> (Callahan, 1993: 169)

First, we need to ask whether such an understanding of death would do the above trick and bring along a meaningful death. Second, is it a good or plausible way to understand death?

Starting with the first question, both suggestions imply an evaluation of dying and death that will make them familiar (which it will be argued is often hedonistically good for us) as well as necessary means (or otherwise intimately linked) to something good. What about the third criterion concerning integration and emotional wholeness? Well, even if our emotions might to some extent respond to rational influence (having rational elements in them), such influencing is not straightforward. Hence, I do not find it unlikely that given such an understanding and evaluation of death, we might still fear death or desperately want to stay alive. If so, such an understanding or evaluation of death would not necessarily bring about greater emotional wholeness or integration between our different inner states and in consequence it is not necessarily conducive to well-being.

Let me make a parallel. We might fully understand that going to a dentist is almost on a par with going to a hospital and hence something familiar to most of us. Moreover, we are likely to evaluate the work of the dentist as a necessary means (though giving rise to pain) to dental health or avoidance of 'dental' suffering. However, even if we admit to all this, we might still fear going to the dentist to the point of actually not going there and instead suffering the worse evil. We might find this irrational and it is, but this is the way we sometimes work. Moreover, this positive understanding and evaluation of the dentist will enhance the inner conflict rather than reduce it. In other words, were we less convinced about the goodness of going to the dentist it would be less of an inner conflict to fear it and avoid it.

Could it be argued that this is a plausible understanding of dying and death? Can we compare death with other events in life (the so-called little deaths) and is it really so that death is a necessary means to some good in life or to a good life? In Callahan we find the following quotation from Arthur C. McGill to illustrate the first point:

> Every time we are sick we hear from within what death shall mean to us personally. Illness is a foretaste of death . . . Every separation from a loved one is a foretaste of death. Every evening, every letting go of the conscious world in sleep is a foretaste of death.
>
> (Callahan 1993: 169)

First, illness is a foretaste of dying rather than of death, if anything. That is, when we are sick we might experience some of the weakness, lack of power and dependency that is associated with dying. However, as long as we have good hopes of total or partial recovery it would seem to be very different from dying and death. When dying (and knowing we are dying) we have no hope of recovery, we know that we will probably get weaker, that our powers will decline even more, that we will become even more dependent until we die and are deprived of any future life. These are essential differences, preventing illness from being a foretaste of death. Moreover, if we take the extinction factor into account illness is even further removed from death. That is to say, illness will generally not imply that I (Lars) am no more. There might be exceptions to this rule, e.g. dementia and other person-changing illnesses, depending on how we view personal identity in relation to these problems. However, even if they are a foretaste of death, they are too good foretastes of death to be usable. That is, if they imply that we exist no more, we cannot benefit from the experience of them, since we are no longer there to benefit. In conclusion, experiencing illnesses will generally not accustom us to death, and when they can, we cannot benefit from that experience.

What about the other comparisons? Death would not be less of a problem

(I gather) if we had good reasons to believe that we would return to the same (or a similar) life after a short while (as with sleep and temporarily saying goodbye to a loved one), or even if we got a somewhat worse life back (as when we lose a loved one for good, by death or separation). Hence, the examples above cannot really be compared with death (and above all with what is problematic in death) and bring familiarity with death along. That is, the problematic thing with death would seem to be just the irreversible loss of life and all the goods of life. To be sure, Callahan (1993: 145) admits that 'There is no way we can envision what it means to be dead.'

What about the idea that death is a necessary means for certain goods in life or even a good life? In another context (Sandman 2001) I have argued that, on the whole, we will live a good life, and (I would say) better life, were there no deaths in our lives. Still, it was admitted that certain goods might be impossible to realize if we do not die. For example, there might be restrictions on having children (and, hence, also grandchildren) due to over-population. Moreover, in Nussbaum (1994) we find a number of examples of possibly good things that we might need to die in order to realize; for example, to sacrifice your life for someone else. Now, if we cannot colonize space we will presumably need to die in order for new generations to be born and, as John Harris (2000) has suggested, choose between children and future life. Here it might be argued that in enabling other generations to be born, we to some extent benefit ourselves and hence it might be in our own interest to die (Seale 1998). Still, in comparison with the value future life might bring us, this value might be outweighed. However, it was argued above that to evaluate one's death as of positive value it might be sufficient to find that it is instrumental in furthering the good of someone else (for example, future generations). That is, that we have to die (and sacrifice our own good) in order to benefit future generations might be the kind of purpose that would give death a meaning to us, with the possible hedonistic benefits resulting from this.

A problem with this argument is that my individual death is not needed to benefit future generations, i.e. my individual death only makes a difference together with the deaths of a large number of other people. Hence, if I were to escape mortality no one would necessarily be harmed as a result of that. Moreover, to some extent this argument depends on the plausibility of the idea that we can harm unborn people by not letting them be born, which is not obvious. However, it also draws on the idea that if we live on we will harm the people existing in the future, when they actually exist.

Walter (1994) relates Victor Frankl's ideas on a good death: I use the remaining days to organize for my loved ones or for the continuation of my projects, and hence benefit other people. However, this is about using my last days in a way that will benefit other people, and does not make death and dying as such meaningful. It would have been better still had I not died and could have continued to care for my loved ones or be involved in these projects in person.

Another reason for the necessity of death in relation to something good found in Callahan is that there is interdependence between good and bad things in life. In other words, the good things need their contrary bad things to be good. He illustrates this idea with a quotation from Hans Jonas: 'the capacity for enjoying the one is the same as that of suffering the other' (Callahan 1993: 170). Even if we admit to this, it does not imply that we actually need the bad things to be present in our lives in order to experience the good things. It is plausible to assume that the capacity to experience (at least some forms of) pleasure is the same as the capacity to experience (at least some forms of) pain or suffering. Still, I do not find it very hard to imagine a world in which there is only pleasure and we only experience pleasure. That is, we have a world in which it is still possible to experience pain, but we do not as a matter of fact have any actual experiences of pain. Now, it might be that we appreciate the pleasure somewhat less in not experiencing any pain and that we would, on the whole, be somewhat better off if we occasionally experienced a little pain to contrast with the pleasure. However, I find it likely that we could do with much less pain than we actually experience today and to be honest I would not mind appreciating pleasure somewhat less if that were the price of removing all pain, especially since most of the pain in the world goes well beyond the need of pain for contrasting effects.

In discussing immortality, I have argued (Sandman 2001) that even if we could have a world in which we did not need to die we would still have the capacity to die. If having this *capacity* is needed to experience some goods, we would surely lose out if we actually 'experienced' death.

Even if these suggestions might convince us that death is indeed meaningful or has a purpose, I do not think they are actually plausible in the sense of being supported by good reasons. If anything, the best bet is the idea about being able to benefit someone else by dying, but that idea suffered from the problem that my individual death might not make much difference.

Elias's meaning

In Norbert Elias's book *The Loneliness of Dying* (1985) there is a short discussion of a meaningful versus a meaningless death that we look at in this section. Consider the following quotation:

> If a thirty-year-old man, the father of two small children and husband of a wife whom he loves and who loves him, is involved in a motorway accident with a driver coming the wrong way, and dies, we say it is a meaningless death . . . because a life that had no relation to that of the affected family, the life of the other driver, at one stroke, as if from

outside and by chance, demolished and destroyed the life, the goals and plans, the happily and firmly rooted feelings of a human being, and thus something that was eminently meaningful for this family . . . If something has . . . a function [with high positive value] for the life of a person and an event furthers or reinforces it, we say it has meaning for her or him. Conversely, when something that has such a function for a person or group ceases to exist, becomes unrealizable or is destroyed, we speak of a loss of meaning.

(Elias 1985: 63)

In essence, Elias seems to claim that if the death of a person has a function or role (according to this person's life projects or goals or values) to fill in that life (or in the lives of other people) it will be meaningful to him. When it does not have such a function or role to fill, it will be a meaningless death. Hence, since being killed in a car accident at the age of thirty does not form part of the life plan or goals of the man in the quotation, his death is meaningless. Perhaps it is even more so, since it seemed to be a result not of the man's own character (or rather character flaws), but of someone else's mistake or recklessness. That is, if a reckless person dies in a car accident, even if not part of his life plans or filling a function in his or other person's life, it would still seem to have some meaning to it according to this idea.

First, if the latter clause is a correct interpretation of what Elias means it would imply that when a habitual smoker dies of lung cancer, this constitutes a more meaningful (and hence better) death than if a health freak dies from the same disease. However, even if it seems true that it is understandable (and hence more meaningful in that sense) if the smoker dies of lung cancer, I see no reason why that death would *ceteris paribus* be better than the death of the non-smoker. Of course, to understand why we die might be comforting for some and in some cases, but in this case when we are, at least partly, responsible for death it would seem to breed strong feelings of regret and anger at our stupidity in smoking.

This is to some extent in line with the rest of Elias's ideas about meaning, i.e. a meaningful death filling a role in the goals and life-plans of the dying person. For someone choosing suicide because of a philosophical conviction or choosing to become a martyr for her beliefs or sacrificing her life to save her children death would be meaningful according to the above. Such a death might be easier to bear to the extent that our emotions align with our convictions about this death. Moreover, it might be a good death according to the waste factor if our death is the fulfilment of an investment in life and there are no other investments that will be wasted as a result of that death.

However, for most deaths and most people this is not the case, i.e. in most cases death is not part of or does not fulfil the life plans or goals of the dying person. Hence, in most cases death would be meaningless according to my interpretation of Elias. Of course, death might in some cases not frustrate any goals or life plans or anything of value in a person's life, and such a death would then be, if not meaningful, at least not meaningless. This is more easily and clearly explained by the deprivation factor and the talk about meaning in such cases would seem rather confusing.

In conclusion, I find that Elias does not seem to add much to the discussion of a good death, except in the few cases where death is in line with or best fulfils the life plans or goals of a person. On the other hand, in these cases Elias seems to say something concerning a good death that is already caught by the waste factor.

Singer's meaning

In Irving Singer's *The Creation of Value* (1996) we find several ideas related to the meaningfulness of death. First is the idea that ends do not necessarily imply that the things they end thereby lose their value. Second, an end can even be what will give these things their value, either because they would lose value if they did not end or because the end is the fulfilment or consummation of these things. Third, death is the correlative or befitting conclusion or result of having lived. Fourth, death is as necessary to life as birth is.

Singer illustrates the first idea with a quotation from George Santayana: 'An invitation to the dance is not rendered ironical because the dance cannot last for ever; the youngest of us and the most vigorously wound up, after a few hours, has had enough of sinuous stepping and prancing' (Singer 1996: 50). It is likely that this is the case with a lot of activities and, I would say, even with life. The fact that life ends does not make the things we do in life meaningless and without value. Even if we will die at some point it will still be valuable to spend the time we have with people we love or enjoy, it will still be valuable to achieve things. So we can agree with Singer (and Santayana) that death does not generally make life meaningless or without value except for the projects that are not fulfilled due to death. However, that does not show that death is therefore meaningful or of value to our lives.

In other words, there seems to be a stronger claim involved in this, namely that if life did not end but went on forever it would lose some or most (or all) of its value. There are several aspects of this idea, the first being that with a finite life we are able to have the motivation to accomplish things: 'In dilatory creatures such as we, it is possible that nothing much would be accomplished without the awareness that time is bounded for us' (Singer 1996: 59). This can be questioned. With unlimited time we would be given opportunity to accomplish a lot more and, besides, we presumably initiate projects mainly because we want to accomplish the goals involved, not because we have little time at our disposal.

Another aspect of this is that if we extend some things eternally, they would become boring and lose much of their value to us; for example, if we danced forever. Here it might be argued that human beings are more imaginative and more plastic than such a view presupposes, even if there might be some truth to such an idea in relation to specific activities. That is, we need not dance our way through life if we do not die; we can vary our lives somewhat more than that.

A third aspect of this second idea is that death might be the consummation or the fulfilment of something and without death it would thereby lose much or its value: 'we can still envisage death as an event that may possibly serve as the appropriate and timely completion of the life that it terminates' (Singer 1996: 58). In the words of Weisman (1973: 376): 'the very last chapter may be why the first chapters were written'. One of the examples Singer gives is of the man fighting in battle and dying when fighting thus. Another could be when the martyr dies for his faith or even more so when Christ dies to fulfil his task of redemption. However, even if there might cases when death is the completion of our life project or one of our life projects, this is not generally so, as was argued in the preceding section on Elias.

Singer's third idea is about death being the natural or correlative and even befitting result of a natural process:

> So . . . may lads and girls, whose hair changes from gold to gray and whose bones turn to dust, undergo death as a natural and correlative result of having lived . . . we eliminate some of its horror if we accept it as the befitting conclusion to a natural process.
>
> (Singer 1996: 59, 60)[6]

Death is obviously the end of a natural process (if life is considered to be a process) and natural in some senses of the word. However, it is not necessarily natural in the sense important here, i.e. the best end to a natural process. Hence, this idea begs the question and no suggestion is given as to why it is befitting that life ends in death. It is simply a brute fact that it does (at least for now) and we need further arguments in order to accept it as something that gives meaning (in the value or purpose sense) to life. In the above it has been argued that death takes value from life.

Finally, it is suggested that birth and death are on par relative to life: 'death is not absurd, just as birth is not. Without the latter, we have no existence; and unless technology can radically alter our current state, the same is true of the former' (Singer 1996: 60). However, this seems patently false. It is of course true that without being born we cannot exist, but *my* death is certainly not necessary in order for *me* to exist. On the contrary, it will rob me of existence. It might be true that my death is in some sense necessary for someone else to exist, but as argued above it is mortality *per se* (given we can only live on this earth) that is necessary for this. It would not make any difference whatsoever if *I* did not die, and if *I* was immortal it would not preclude anyone else from living.

In conclusion, Singer does not seem to add any convincing arguments not already dealt with for why death should or could be considered meaningful (i.e. of value or fulfilling a purpose) to us.

Summary

It has been argued that the interpretation of meaningful death that has the best chance of being successful in making for a better death is to find death to be of positive instrumental value to something or someone, and for our emotions in the face of death to align themselves with this understanding. If death is found to have meaning there is a good chance of dying being somewhat less hedonistically troublesome. Here it is important to point out that it is our subjective view on whether death has value or not that is important, not the actual value it has.

To the extent that such an evaluation will be successful in having us conclude that death has meaning, it has to have a certain degree of plausibility (even if it does not have to be true). In the analysis of a number of different suggestions for what might make us find death meaningful it was argued that the most plausible suggestions were the idea about our death being necessary to benefit other and future people and the idea about death as the fulfilment of our life projects or goals. However, in the latter case it was questioned whether such an idea had any great relevance, since we found it reasonable to assume that the number of cases of such deaths is few. In relation to the former case, it was argued that even if mortality probably is essential to the good of future generations, my individual death is not. Hence it might be difficult to convince myself that my death is actually needed and has a purpose.

Normative aspects of a meaningful death

Since meaning in the sense of value and purpose to life is at the heart of the goal of palliative care (see Chapter 7) it is essential that professional carers try to enable dying patients and their close ones to live their last days as valuably or meaningfully as possible. That is, patients and close ones must be enabled to do the things they take pleasure in, or the things they desire or that add to their objective list values.

However, when we look at death as such for the dying patient, it is more doubtful whether it is possible to find death to be of value or to have a good purpose. Of course, normally carers should support whatever meaning the patient takes comfort in, even if the carer does not find any real support for such a meaning to be found in death. On the other hand, if the patient is adamant about the meaning she subscribes to being in accordance with the way things really are, carers will have a reason to try to be as sincere about this as possible.

What about those who do not find any meaning? I believe we should be careful in trying to convince the patient about a meaning that we do not ourselves believe and that might not be in line with what the patient really believes. Perhaps death is actually meaningless in the sense of having no good purpose and we should instead make things as good as possible given such a view.

When carers are helping the patient and his or her close ones to a meaningful death, they cannot be obliged to risk their own good life. As mentioned above, this is, to some extent, dependent on things like whether carers have access to counselling and are well prepared to deal with these kinds of situations. However, this does not mean that the carers only have to accept a death and dying that is meaningful to them, i.e. when talking about risk to their own good life, only the kind of risk with long-lasting consequences that cannot be relieved by counselling or a short perod of rest should be taken into account. A check should be made of the care culture. Is there an established view of what meaning death has within the care context and to what extent will carers influence the patient and their close ones to adopt such a view?

A dignified death

In the discussion of palliative care and within palliative care we often find the idea that death should be dignified or that we should be enabled to die with dignity[7] (see Sandman 2003). 'Dignity' is obviously a so-called 'thick' concept, i.e. a concept which involves both evaluative and descriptive aspects. The evaluative aspects are generally positive and 'dignity' is sometimes used synonomously with 'good' (especially in care contexts). However, the descriptive aspects of the concept are less clear or transparent. It is only to the extent that the concept is well defined and precise that we can use it as a guiding concept in relation to good dying. Here we might identify some different problems. First, there are at least two different but related concepts in use, dignity and human dignity, and the relationship between them is not fully clear. Second, these meanings can be given different normative and evaluative implications for dying. Third, it is not exactly clear how we would qualify to have dignity in any of the above senses. In Saunders and Baines (1983) it is even claimed that such confusion concerning the concept of dignity should lead us to avoid it within the palliative context. However, let us see if we can make some sense of this concept and how it might be relevant to a good dying.

As indicated in the introductory remarks it is important to distinguish between *human dignity* (see Sandman 2002 for a further discussion of this) and dignity in a more general sense, what we might call *contingent dignity*. While human dignity is supposed to be something that belongs to all human beings, contingent dignity is something we have due to certain features, more or less deep and not necessarily common to all humans. Hence, if the talk of dignity implies that we are formal and controlled we obviously talk of dignity in the contingent sense, as in the following newspaper quotation from Walter (1994: 19), reporting from the funeral of a three-year old IRA victim: 'The grief finally became too much today. Despite the barriers of dignity and pride that Wilf and Marie Ball had tried to erect around their son's senseless death, the emotions broke through.' The idea about human dignity being central to palliative care is obvious in the Swedish context. The Swedish Parliamentary Report on Palliative Care states:

> Palliative care should rest on ethical premises based on the principle of equal human (innate) dignity . . . Human (innate) dignity is tied to the human being as a person, disregarding any functions or features this person might have. All human beings have an equal dignity (value).
>
> (SOU 2001: 53, 54, my translation)

Ideas about contingent dignity would also seem to be central within palliative care.[8]

When speaking in terms of human dignity it is self-evident that we are making both evaluative and normative claims. We claim that humans have a high (or even absolute) value and imply that this should guide the way we treat them. Similarly, the contingent dignity implies a high value in the bearer and that this has implications for how we should treat him or her.

Human dignity

Two questions need to be answered in relation to human dignity and its role within palliative care. First, why do we have this high value? Second, what does it imply for palliative care if humans have this high value?

A preliminary answer to the first of these questions would be that we simply have this value in being human. This answer does not seem wholly satisfactory, especially not in the wake of evolutionary biology, secularization and the discussion on animal rights. That is, to claim that humans have a special moral or evaluative standing in creation just for being humans would seem to be a case of so-called speciesism. Hence, to be intellectually satisfactory we need another answer to this question that includes all humans (and perhaps other animals).[9]

There are a number of suggestions, which all suffer from the problem of not being inclusive enough, i.e. having the implication that not all humans have this dignity. Examples are that we are autonomous or self-conscious (Bayertz 1996). Obviously not all human beings are autonomous or self-conscious even if we have very free criteria for these features. For example, would newborns, severely demented people or severely mentally impaired people fall outside these criteria if there should be anything to the idea of autonomy or self-consciousness.

There are, however, some suggestions as to how one could save the idea of human dignity (see Sandman 2002 for a more thorough discussion of these). First, it could be claimed that it is enough if the species has these character-istics even if not every single individual has them. Second, it could be claimed that it is enough if we have the potential to have these character-istics, even if they are not actually instantiated. Third, we could base the dignity in something that also includes other (so-called lower) creatures.

When we focus on people at the end of life it seems that only the last route would be open. One suggestion would be to base our dignity in our ability to experience suffering and well-being, an ability we share with a number of other creatures. This would also be a way to include those groups mentioned above, i.e. newborns and severely demented people, since they do have the ability to experience suffering. Perhaps this suggestion would still be prob-lematic, since our ability to suffer differs from person to person, something that is not in line with an equal human dignity. Hence, we obviously still have a problem in providing a base for an equal and high human dignity satisfactorily.

Another important question is why this idea about an equal and high human dignity is normatively important for palliative care. One central implication is that it helps us to ground an equal and impartial treatment of human beings, not taking into consideration features that are not nor-matively relevant (Tännsjö 1998b). If we all have the same value and moral treatment is founded in such a value, it seems to imply that we should be treated in an equal and impartial (though not necessarily identical) manner. Hence, when passing moral judgements on how to treat other people, we only let things that are morally relevant come into play. This will then give us a framework for palliative care, but not really give us any substantial ideas as to what to do. First we need to clarify what is and what is not morally relevant. Moreover, if we have to assume such a value (unfounded), why not assume equal and impartial treatment without taking the detour around human dignity?

Could it be that the idea about a high and equal human value has other normative implications that make it essential? One such implication could be that no effort should be spared in saving such a life, since the loss would be very high indeed. This is, however, not in line with the values of palliative care, which does not advocate prolongation of life at any cost (see, for example, WHO 1990).

Another implication would be that if humans have this value, other people should treat them as valuables, i.e. 'handle them with care'. Why do we normally treat valuables with care? First, we might risk their value by damaging them. Second, they might deserve such a treatment due to the value they have. The first idea does not seem relevant here, since a premise is that we cannot lose the value we have (at least not as long as we are still alive). It is of course obvious that we might hurt people or cause them suffering in different ways in treating them badly. Still, to me it seems obvious that we should avoid treating them thus because we cause them suffering, not because they have a certain value.

When we come to the second idea it presupposes that we have some idea about what a human being of high value deserves and that is supposedly connected to what is good for her, i.e it is related to the question 'What is a good life?' Perhaps this idea about human dignity could be the foundation on which to base a norm about all human beings deserving a good life and hence also that for making this the overall goal of palliative care (which it is in many formulations) (Sandman 2003). This still does not give us any concrete guidance as to what good palliative care should imply.

A conclusion would hence be that human dignity could, perhaps, function as a foundation for a general goal of providing good life to people in the palliative phase. However, we should often use a more concrete discourse in which we talk in terms of equality and impartiality and about realizing a good life for patients, at least if the concepts we use should have some action-guiding role.

Contingent dignity

If we instead look at how contingent dignity could be relevant for dying the good death, we can distinguish a number of different uses and meanings in the concept of dignity (where some are more closely related to the ideas about what grounds the human dignity). First, we can have certain personality traits or character traits; for example, that we are solemn or controlled (Callahan 1993; Walter 1994; Kolnai 1995). Second, we can have a certain social standing or role in society – the dignity of being a bishop or a professor. Third, we can have a certain effect on other people – that we inspire awe or respect in them (Sandman 2001). Fourth, we can have a certain way to relate to ourselves – in having self-respect or self-esteem (Momeyer 1988; Sandman 2001; Nordenfelt 2003).

Outside the health-care context (for example, in novels) dignity is normally associated with a number of character traits or a certain way to behave (as was seen in the quotation from Walter 1994 above):

the qualities of composure, calmness, restraint, reserve, and emotions and passions subdued and securely controlled without being negated or dissolved . . . qualities of distinctness, delimitation, and distance; of something that conveys the idea of being intangible, invulnerable, inaccessible to destructive or corruptive or subversive interference.

(Kolnai 1995: 56)

Richard Momeyer also claims that dignity in this sense is basically an aristocratic feature, something that will distinguish between different people: 'The Latin word *dignitas* denotes honorableness, worth, excellence, and desert; it applies to persons of high rank or estate (dignitaries). Such persons are expected to have a nobility of manner or style' (Momeyer 1988: 71). It seems that Daniel Callahan subscribes, more or less, to this picture of what dignity implies.[10] Consider the following quotation from Leon R. Kass in Callahan's discussion of dignity:

It is a term of distinction; dignity is not something which, like a nose or a navel, is to be expected or found in every living human being. Dignity is, in principle, aristocratic – that is inescapable, quite apart from the way one might specify the content of excellence or distinction. It follows that dignity, thus understood, cannot be demanded or claimed; for it cannot be provided and it is not owed. One has no more *right* to dignity – and hence to dignity in death – than one has to beauty or courage or wisdom, desirable though these may be.

(Callahan 1993: 147)

This notion of dignity is different from the above, more inclusive, human dignity. As explicitly claimed in the latter quotation, dignity is here a sign of distinction and excellence, of rising above the mass or herd. Consequently, only the few will presumably be able to die a dignified death. The world might be a place where it is difficult and only the very few will be blessed with a good death, even if this is not in line with the idea about human dignity. Hence we need to ask whether dignity, thus understood, really makes for a better death. This is discussed in Chapter 4, where the issue of controlling problematic emotions and thoughts is dealt with, and where the conclusion is that the support for this stoical ideal is equivocal. This support could be even more doubtful when dignity implies more than just controlling problematic emotions and thoughts, but actually controlling all emotions and thoughts.

Moreover, if taking into account what a dignified death in this sense normally implies for the external environment I find even less support for the idea. That is, traditionally (in our cultural context) a dignified death is silent, surrounded by lit candles and grave and serious persons dressed in dark colours giving exalted and exalting speeches. These people do not display feelings, or they display them in a controlled way; they do not allow themselves to become pathetic and keep their distance. For example, Nuland (1993: 191) claims that 'When a person is dying, the walls of the room make up a chapel in which you only trod in silenced awe.' It is not obvious (to me, at least) that this is a better death than a death surrounded by a bunch of noisy people, talking and joking and drinking, dressed in whatever they fancy, openly displaying their feelings; especially if this has been what the dying person has enjoyed or what is associated with a special occasion for him. It has sometimes been claimed that this dignified attitude of people visiting and working with dying people results in the environment of the dying person being characterized by death long before the person has actually died. This is also a reason, voiced in conversations, why people tend to shun special institutions for dying people. That is to say, they risk 'experiencing' death before it actually happens, due to the funeral-like environment.

Even if the above quotation from Callahan indicates that dignity is something we cannot acquire to any large extent (see the comments on beauty), other quotations give the general impression that we can acquire dignity in the above sense or (at least) act and behave as if we have dignity. People who are not, normally, dignified might obviously act in a dignified way on special occasions, such as a funeral: 'Our dignity will stem from the way we come to understand and master that loss [of control], not from the loss itself.' Later in the text Callahan writes: 'Mastery requires that our interior self be in charge of itself, even when death is coming and control over the body has been, as it must be, lost . . . Dignity is not something given to us. We create our own dignity' (Callahan 1993: 147).

Even if this will make it somewhat less exclusive to die a dignified death, I find the same conclusions as before applicable here. That is, I see no reasons why acting and behaving with dignity would generally make for a better death. The main reasons why such dignity would make for a better death is, as is elaborated in Chapter 4, that it might be instrumental in getting what we want or enjoy or in implying less strain to relationships. But even if this might apply to self-control over problematic emotions and cognitions to some extent, it would not seem generally applicable to all the above features of dignity. It is as likely to be detrimental to relationships, since dignity here implies a certain emotional distance and close relationships do (as the name signals) require a certain amount of closeness and intimacy that the dignified person might have a difficulty achieving. A sign of exaltation is obviously that other people cannot reach you or are kept at a distance. Moreover, from a hedonistic and desire fulfilment approach it is not generally the case that we benefit from being dignified in this sense. I would even take it that a lot of people may suffer from having to be dignified at the end of life in the same way as we might suffer or, at least, feel inconvenient on very solemn or formal occasions. Perhaps this is to some extent related to class. Lawton (2000) found that people's class backgound tends to linger on in dying, and working-class patients preferred sharing a room with other dying patients and middle-class patients preferred the privacy of a single room. Here some of the comments indicate that one of the reasons for the middle-class patients wanting a single room was dignity-related in this aristocratic sense: 'the other patients [in the wards] used to drive me mad . . . all their menial conversation and inane questions' (Lawton 2000: 169).

Hence, to the extent that you already have a dignified personality it is likely that a dignified death in which that personality is not compromised will be a better death than a death in which you are urged or forced to act in a way not in line with your personality, especially since you are not likely to be able to change personality within the short time left. However, for the same reasons as above it is doubtful whether it will make for a better death if people in the vicinity of the dying person act dignified (unless it is part of their personality or we are dealing with a dignified person).

A possible reason in favour of dignity in this sense is that acting thus will not make other people feel inconvenient or awkward, which is good on a hedonistic account. But perhaps we should not spare people inconvenience or awkwardness in being confronted with death, since death is generally bad. Besides, people might also be uncomfortable with dignified people. Moreover, if people are uncomfortable with people acting in a way that is on the whole not problematic, we should probably ignore that – as we should ignore people getting upset over homosexuals or policewomen or whatever.

In conclusion, I find it doubtful that this aristocratic notion of dignity would generally make for a better death if implemented, whether on behalf of the dying person or on behalf of people in the vicinity. However, people already aristocratically dignified might be better off if they continue to be dignified in death, though they might have been, on the whole, better off had they not had such a personality or character.

The idea of dignity in relation to certain social roles or standings in society is obviously closely related to the above aristocratic notion, i.e. traditionally we did not talk of the dignity of a worker and when we do it is a matter of trying to conquer this aristocratic notion. Normally when we use the concept of dignity in relation to social roles we also (I think) refer to characteristics like the above – a bishop should be grave and serious rather than frivolous and silly.

This idea about a certain dignity related to certain social roles conflicts with the idea about human dignity, i.e. since dignity implies having a certain value, a bishop would have the value of being human together with the value of being a bishop, and hence score better in the value league. This is something that is not in line with the idea about human dignity, where value is supposed to be equally distributed among human beings.

Moreover, even if my position in society might influence what I enjoy or what I desire when I am about to die (see the comments about class above, Lawton 2000), this position *per se* would not seem to have anything to do with whether I get a good death or not. And from a normative perspective, it seems obvious that it should not play a role in what care to receive other than indirectly, i.e. in that we take the person's desires into account. These desires may of course be related to the person's position in society, or they may not be so related. To a large extent it seems that the dignity character-istics associated with having a certain role or position in society have eroded or lost most of their content. Bishops and professors come in all forms nowadays. In conclusion, this aspect of dignity would not seem to be relevant in the context of good dying and death.

The third idea, also somewhat related to the aristocratic idea, is the idea about being awe-inspiring. The relation is, however, contingent, since we might be awe-inspiring even with another personality than the above aristocratic one. Still, since we traditionally have associated these features with a high standing in society the above personality is likely to be one of the personalities that are awe-inspiring. This idea also draws on the idea about human dignity, since one of the inferences we could take from the idea about human dignity is that we should not treat someone with a high value in any way we like. However, here this idea rests on actual features of the person, not in an abstract notion of the value of this person.

When we are dependent on other people in dying, we might actually benefit from being awe-inspiring. That is, if someone is awe-inspiring it normally implies something about the way we approach her and treat her. We assume a certain carefulness in how we approach her, we assume a certain attitude of wonder towards her and there is a certain resistance in approaching someone who is awe-inspiring. Hence, we do not treat some-one who is awe-inspiring in any way we like, and it would not even come to mind to treat her thus. People who are awe-inspiring are likely to have it their way and to be taken seriously. Moreover, people will generally be careful not to cause them distress or disturb them and they will be careful not to neglect them. This would presumably be good for us on any account of good. The example *par excellence* of someone who is awe-inspiring is God, and we might imagine how we would approach someone who is omnipotent and omniscient. As the illustration in the Bible would have it, we would not approach such a creature lightly.

A problem is that not all people (or perhaps not even most people) do inspire awe in us when in their normal situation and especially not when they are dying. As Lawton (2000) vividly describes in the report of her observational study of palliative care, the bodily decay of dying patients is not something that makes them awe-inspiring; if anything they might rather be viewed as non-persons. Hence, few would be fortunate enough to benefit from dignity in this way. Still, it might be the ideal way to be at the end of life, if or when dependent on other people.

Further problems with being awe-inspiring are the same as those pre-sented above regarding aristocratic dignity, i.e. that we would seem to risk loneliness in making other people reluctant to get close to us. Other people would keep their distance from us or would not dare to speak their minds to us. However, that might be to overstate the problem, since it is not difficult to imagine that someone who is awe-inspiring has intimate personal relationships. It is the more temporary relations he or she has that will not easily develop into close ones, i.e. the care personnel will not get close to such a person.

In conclusion, to have dignity in the sense of being awe-inspiring, whether that implies having the above aristocratic features or other features, would seem beneficial to some extent given that we are involved in dependency relations. However, besides the obvious problem that not all people are awe-inspiring, especially when dying, on the whole we might risk losing out on both hedonistic benefits in general and relational goods in particular by being such persons.

Let us move on to a perspective on contingent dignity that could, in distinction to the three above, be somewhat more evenly distributed among human beings. As a starting point consider the following quotation from Momeyer:

> In our more democratic age . . . 'dignity' has been spread about (some no doubt would say diluted), so that in certain crucial respects it is held to belong to every person. The most vital dimensions of dignity . . . seem to be the following:
>
> 1 *Consciousness and Rationality* . . . Consciousness and the capacity for rationality constitute human dignity in the most generic sense, for all those we would be prepared to call persons . . .
> 2 *Self-determination* (Autonomy) . . . The opportunity to make one's own choices and to implement these without interference by others . . .
> 3 *Bodily Integrity*. Well enculturated human being typically place enormous value upon how they physically appear to others . . .
> 4 *Self-esteem*. How one feels about one's self is an important aspect of human dignity.
>
> (Momeyer 1988: 71–3)

Here Momeyer is talking in terms of human dignity, and this concept is obviously less exclusive than the aristocratic one. However, since the focus here is on contingent dignity, I will deal with Momeyer's suggestion as saying something about one type of contingent dignity; and it seems the essential part here is self-respect or self-esteem.

If dignity is about the value a human being has, contingent or not, it is obviously closely related to the ideas about self-respect or self-esteem, since they say both something about how I view or relate to myself and what value I ascribe to myself. We find this supported in other contexts as well:

> Dignity has been defined as having a sense of personal worth. The dignity of one person is not absolute, but depends on the way that people behave towards that person . . . The role of professional carers must be to enhance a person's sense of dignity at all times.
>
> (Finlay 1996: 69; see also Nordenfelt 2003)

Since it is difficult to imagine that it would not negatively affect our well-being or that it would have any instrumentally beneficial effects to score low on self-esteem, this would be strongly supported by the hedonistic approach, and by the desire fulfilment approach, ignoring those with a masochistic bent or who desire to punish themselves. If we bring in the restrictions of the desire fulfilment approach, we might even get universal support for the idea that self-esteem would add to the value of life. That is, desiring to be useless or worthless or desiring things that imply that we are useless would presumably be one of the things that would be considered objectively undesirable, or the result of adaptive desires. We might of course desire to be useless or worthless if we do not approve of the standards of society, but it is more difficult to imagine that we would want to be useless or worthless if we do approve of them.

With an objective list approach we would get a similar result, at least considering the instrumental value of having high self-esteem for things like achievements and relationships. However, a possible problem here is the idea of being in contact with reality. We should only estimate ourselves to have the value we actually have (given the character of our lives) and neither exaggerate it nor underestimate it. Hence, reality contact would have us acknowledge that we are worthless if indeed we are (given the proper standards for this, which might not be the socially established or approved standards). If we find this unacceptable, we might have to admit to the restriction on this idea that we need not acknowledge what is a bad situation for us. Or we might salvage our self-esteem in claiming that no person is worthless, since just being a person (or a human being) has a certain high value. However, if this is not all there is to self-esteem, and it is not, since we normally do not take pride in or esteem ourselves for just being human, it might not do much good if we cannot point to some other feature of life that will actually make it valuable. In comparison with other people we will still be of less value, since we only have what all the others have and do not have what they have on top of this. Disregarding reality contact, dignity in terms of self-esteem or self-respect would have strong support in making for a good or better death.

How should we view the rest of Momeyer's list or, revealing my views on his suggestions, what can influence our self-esteem or self-respect? That is, I find it reasonable to view Momeyer's list as things that might, for many people, influence their self-esteem, self-respect or self-identity (which would seem to be related to what value we place on ourselves). First, without consciousness and rationality, we are not able to have any views what-soever on who we are and what value we are in possession of. Hence, the first item on the list would be a necessary criterion for having self-esteem or self-respect. However, here it is important to be clear that we can still die a good death, at least on the well-being approach, if we lack rationality and at least some aspects of consciousness. Moreover, sometimes the best death is to move into terminal unconsciousness or even get rid of consciousness altogether (i.e. die). In other words, self-esteem is only important for those who are able to have high esteem for themselves.

Moving on, for a lot of people (at least in our cultural context) self-determination is vital to their self-identity and hence also to being able to have high self-esteem. In Lawton (2000) one of the conclusions is that loss of self-determination, at least in the sense of losing one's ability to perform what one decides upon but also in the sense of influencing the life around them, is detrimental to people's self-identity and the value they place on themselves. This is even more the case for the loss of bodily integrity where the 'unbounded' body, in Lawton's words, not only affects the dying person's own self-image or self-identity but leads to people in the vicinity treating the dying person as a non-person (Lawton 2000). This is also related to self-determination in a way, since people lose the ability to control the bodily functions they normally could control. Consider the following description of Annie, one of the hospice patients: 'every time she attempted to get out of bed and stand up, diarrhoea and urine would pour straight out of her body' (Lawton 2000: 125).

Lawton also observes how the loss of bodily integrity affects another essential aspect of self-identity and self-esteem, the dying person's relation-ships. Other patients distance themselves from the person who has lost his bodily integrity, and the dying person's close ones cannot maintain the kind of relationship they used to. For example, one of the reasons why patients were admitted was that their close ones could no longer handle the odour of the patients in their home (Lawton 2000). Bodily decay will influence rela-tionships in yet other ways, i.e. in that dying people are no longer able to do the things they used to do in the relationship, such as visit common meeting places or show affection.

Hence, even if we might have an idealized view of self-esteem in the sense that we should be able to find ourselves valuable in almost any circum-stances just for being the people we are, this is indeed idealized and rests on a view of persons that presupposes them to be something almost spiritual, with no real characteristics. It is more plausible to have a more down-to-earth view on persons, where we are the persons we are due to the actual characterstics we have, i.e. things like our bodily appearance, our mental make-up, our actions and decisions. Moreover, we place the value we assign to ourselves in having these characteristics, and when we lose them that will affect the value we assign to ourselves. In other words, it will affect our self-identity and self-esteem. Here it is of course important to point out that the making of our identity is not something done in isolation from other people, and the social context will give us clues to who we are and to what value we have; and it seems the features discussed here are given an important standing in our society. However, we might find self-esteem in having other features and should be careful about viewing self-determination, bodily integrity or close relationships as essential for high self-esteem for all people.

Summary

In this section it has been argued that the concept of dignity can be distinguished in at least two different categories: the idea of human dignity as equal and belonging to all human beings, and the idea of dignity in terms of having certain character traits or features or behaving in specific ways. I concluded that the idea of human dignity suffered from two problems in relation to a dignified death. First is the obvious problem of grounding this dignity in something that is ethically and value relevant and that is neither too exclusive nor too inclusive. Second, accepting this idea, we are given almost no clues as to what it implies for the content of a good death, even if it might tell us that all human beings should have a good death or that the death of a human being is always a great loss or bad. Hence, the idea of human dignity does not seem very useful in relation to the concept of a good death.

Looking at what dignity in the contingent sense implies, it was concluded that dignity in the traditional and aristocratic sense does not generally make for a better death unless we have been a dignified person in that sense all through life. It might have some benefits but it also has obvious drawbacks in terms of lack of intimacy and in losing out on possible hedonistic benefits. Moreover, it will make dignity in death an overly exclusive feature. Nor did dignity in the social role sense have much going for it. A related idea is that of being awe-inspiring and it was concluded that this has some benefits to the extent that we are dependent on other people in dying, since it is likely to prevent some of the risks attached to such dependency becoming realized. Still, as with the aristocratic idea it implies a certain formality in how we are treated, something that is normally associated with a hedonistic cost and a risk of distance in relationships. Hence, on the whole we might be worse off for being awe-inspiring in dying and death. Moreover, few people will be awe-inspiring in dying, owing to their weakened condition.

Finally, dignity as self-respect or self-esteem was explored and was found to have strong support for making for a good dying, to the extent that we are in the position to have self-esteem. Self-esteem, it was concluded, is for a lot of people related to things like being self-determined, having bodily integrity and upholding close relationships – changes in these characteristics will often affect people's self-esteem.

Consequently, the most important aspect of dignity is self-esteem, and to the extent that a dignified death implies a death with maintained or even enhanced self-esteem, a dignified death is a good or better death. However, since dignity is a notoriously unclear concept, with a number of different connotations, it would perhaps be better to talk about what makes for a dignified death in concrete terms (see Sandman 2003 for a discussion of this); that is, to talk in terms of self-esteem, aristocratic features or whatever aspect of dignity we refer to and evaluate these according to their own merits, not according to whether they make us dignified in death or not.

Normative aspects of a dignified death

Carers should support the opinions of patients when they concern what it is to die with dignity. More generally, carers should be careful to strengthen or at least not weaken the self-esteem or self-respect of the patient, to the extent possible given the dying person's condition. However, carers should be careful not to present an overly idealistic view on what the person might find self-esteem in when he or she cannot be thus convinced. In such a case, it seems proper to confirm the person's own views about his or her condition.

Even if dignity is associated with having death induced for some patients, carers cannot be called upon to break the law in order for a person to die with dignity. Hence, as long as it is legally prohibited to provide euthanasia, carers are not required to aid patients in this, even if this is according to the patients' views on a death with dignity.

Moreover, we have to be attentive about what the philosophy of the palliative care context signals in terms of what a dignified death is in order to allow the patient's own views on this to be accorded with; and we should also be attentive about our own opinions on what a dignified death is, especially if these opinions or this philosophy are supportive of a view on dignity that is experienced as repressive by the patient.

Conclusions and relevance to palliative care

In this chapter we have discussed whether there are certain global features a death should have in order to become a good death. In other words, are there general characterstics we could give a good death that would be part of or the whole of a good death?

First, we discussed the idea of dying a consistent death, and it was argued that to the extent that we still maintain the wants and ideals we have had throughout our lives, we have reason to die a consistent death. Consistency as such does not have any strong support. It may demonstrate that we normally do not change much over time and hence if we are given the opportunity to lead the same kind of life we have lived before, most of us will benefit from this. This is of course relevant to palliative care, since we find norms like 'living until you die' and 'remaining the same person as before' within the palliative care philosophy, and we need to be aware of the extent to which this will actually bring value to the dying person. However, in palliative care we are dying, with all that dying might imply in terms of changes and losses. Hence, we cannot take for granted that a dying that is consistent with the rest of the person's life will necessarily benefit him. It should depend on whether the dying person still wants to live the kind of life he used to live.

Second, we discussed the idea of a meaningful death and it was argued that if a meaningful death should mean something other than just a good death, we should focus on the extent to which death fulfils an important purpose (has positive instrumental value) in our lives. None of the suggestions discussed was found to have much support and we ended up with the conclusion that in the cases when our death actually benefits someone else our death can be said to be meaningful, and individual deaths do not generally do that. When my death is the fulfilment of my projects my death can be said to be meaningful, which again is not the case for most people. This is relevant to palliative care, as such care has the objective of dealing with the existential problems of the dying patient or, in other words, helping the dying patient to make sense of death or find some purpose in death. If most of the suggestions for what makes death meaningful are not relevant or reasonable to the dying patient we face the question of what we are allowed to do in order to find a sense that will actually comfort the dying patient. Perhaps we should be open to the fact that there might not actually be any sense or meaning at all in the death of the patient and instead try to find comfort in what is still left in life.

Third, we discussed the idea of a dignified death and it was argued that the multifaceted concept of dignity should be replaced by the more concrete descriptions of what we mean when we talk in terms of dignity. A number of different meanings of dignity were explored and the one found to have the strongest support in relation to a good dying or death was dignity in terms of self-esteem. The more aristocratic notions were found to be problematic in different ways, mainly since they are related to a stoic and controlled way of handling death and dying that is not necessarily in the best interest of the dying person. The notion of human dignity was found to be more or less useless as action-guiding in relation to palliative care due to the number of possible interpretations and also due to the problem of actually founding the notion in an acceptable way. In relation to palliative care dignity is relevant for several reasons. First, it is a concept that is commonly used, but seldom explicated, within palliative care and we need to be clear about what we mean when we claim that palliative care should lead to a dignified death for the dying patient. Second, the interpretation of dignity given support in this context, i.e. self-esteem, seems to be an important aspect or precondition of actually being able to remain a person and continue to live until one dies, and not facing social death before biological death.

Notes

1 See Loewy and Springer Loewy (2000: 3), where diachronic consistency is advocated, but with the proviso that most lives *are* diachronically consistent.
2 See, for example, Gordijn and Janssens (2000: 44), who argue along these lines.
3 I owe this example to Gunnar Eckerdal.
4 See Daniel (1996) for a similar discussion of rectifying in death.
5 See also Loewy and Springer Loewy (2000: 19–20), Larsson (1984), Beck-Friis (1990), Gunnars and Borgenhammar (both in Beck-Friis and Strang 1995) and Twycross (1995), some of whom refer to the ideas of Frankl (1963).
6 See also Weisman (1973: 367).
7 See, for example, SOU (2001) and Janssens (2001), who refers to a European study within the PALLIUM project (palliative care ethics) where 96.2 per cent of the palliative carers judged 'dignity' a central concept within palliative care.
8 See, for example, Kübler-Ross (1969, 1974), Feigenberg (1979), SOU (1979), Beck-Friis (1990), McNamara *et al.* (1994) and Hanratty and Higginson (1994).
9 Here it could be argued that if this value belongs to more creatures than humans, we should also be interested in their dignified death. However, I will ignore that aspect in this context. This is not because I find it unimportant, but because this book deals with palliative care for humans.
10 We also find this kind of 'proper behaviour' in death described in Glaser and Strauss (1965: Chapter 5).

4 Facing death

Following the discussion of overall aspects of a good dying in Chapter 3, this chapter focuses on different attitudes to death and dying and features of death and dying. In other words, it discusses the best way to face death, whether we will be better at facing death having experienced the death of others, whether we have reason to adopt certain cognitive and emotional attitudes to death when dying and if so whether we should display these attitudes or not in dying. Finally, are there some sufferings we have reason to accept in dying rather than get rid of?

Acquaintance with death

In the literature and discussion on good death it is often argued that death is something we avoid getting acquainted with, something we avoid talking about nowadays and hence something we are less familiar with compared to our forebears.[1] Death has become taboo, in modern society and, it is argued, was historically more familiar and less taboo, in that it was a 'routine part of daily life' (Callahan 1993: 26) and 'never far away' (Ariés 1981: 15). This has been questioned by several writers on the issue of good death, who argue (convincingly) that the issue of death has seen a revival and that death is treated not as a taboo in our society but as something private (see, for example, Walter 1994; Seale 1998).

Regardless of whether death is taboo or not in our society, we might still discuss whether we have general reasons to get acquainted with death to prepare for our own death or for the death of others. In this section we focus on whether getting acquainted with death and dying, so to speak in the flesh, would be beneficial to us. In the next section we take a look at the related idea of whether talking and thinking about our own death would be beneficial to us, what has been called awareness of death.

Even if death is not actually taboo in our society, it seems reasonable to claim that people nowadays do not encounter dying people in the flesh as often as our ancestors did. When they do encounter dying people, it is often rather late in life. What could account for this? Two factors seem to play an important role here: first, the medicalization of death, i.e. dying and death is now within the domain of the medical professions and takes place, to a large extent, within medical institutions; second, the development of a welfare society with its lowering of the infant mortality rates and its increase in the average life expectancy of people.[2] That is, historically, before we had reached the age of 20 we would probably have experienced the death of our grandparents, the death of some of our siblings, perhaps the death of our parents and perhaps even the death of some of our own children. Moreover, since people shared everyday life to a greater extent and there were few if any alternatives to dying at home, it was hard to avoid the death of someone in the vicinity. However, we should not allow people to die in early age just to ensure that we are better acquainted with death, even though Norbert Elias expresses some doubt as to this in the following quotation, in which he also vividly describes what was at stake:

> life in this medieval society was shorter, the dangers less controllable, dying often more painful, the sense of guilt and fear of punishment after death an official doctrine; but, for better or for worse, the participation of others in an individual's death was far more normal.
>
> (Elias 1985: 16)

Hence, what we could do to encounter more deaths, and something that would be ethically more acceptable, is to try to encounter death when it occurs, i.e. when we are no longer able to fence it off with better health care or other measures. This is something that could be done by visiting dying people in hospitals but we might also, to the extent we find it beneficial, encourage acquaintance with death by allowing more people to die at home. However, I would say that there are more pressing reasons for allowing people to die at home, i.e. that people actually want to die at home. Still, to judge whether greater familiarity with death would be something worth experiencing, we need to know why it is beneficial to us, if indeed it is.

More generally, why is it beneficial to be familiar in advance with something that is generally bad or dreadful for us, once we encounter this ourselves? Let me start by making a parallel with a public presentation. The first time you give a public presentation (in school or wherever) it is probably experienced as rather scary; you feel awkward and uneasy in the situation. You are nervous and do not know how best to present your material, which is likely to affect your performance. After having given a number of presentations you might find yourself more at ease, you realize that it is not that scary and your performance is enhanced. Being acquainted with situations that are initially negatively valued may hence influence how we perceive and handle such situations later on. In many cases the result will be that we experience these situations as less troublesome, one reason being that what we know we can control.

Is death on a par with public presentation when it comes to the benefits of familiarity? Getting acquainted with public presentations in order to experience them as less problematic will normally require acquaintance from a first person perspective, i.e. actually training to give the presentation yourself. However, when it comes to death and dying, acquaintance can mainly be had from a third person perspective. That is, we can encounter the dying and death of other people. Of course, we can encounter what we believe to be, but which is not, our own dying a number of times and we can be familiar with some of the aspects that might be problematic in dying. But apart from being different from actually getting acquainted with one's own dying and death, in this context it is mainly a third person acquaintance with death that is advocated. In other words, we would die a better death ourselves if we frequently encountered the deaths of others. So, let us focus on the third person perspective since the rather few cases of first person acquaintance with dying and death would seem a bit peripheral to this discussion.

Value to the dying person

We should look at public presentations from the perspective of being a spectator watching a number of such presentations before doing one's first and only public presentation. Listening to other people's presentations does not generally make it easier for us to present something or make us better presenters, even if we might get a few good tips (from both a good presentation and a bad one). However, this might not be all that easy to put into practice when actually doing a presentation on our own. As most of us know, we might listen to an abundance of confident and relaxed public presentations but still find it very unpleasant to give a presentation of our own (and in this context it is implied that we are not given the opportunity to train to give such a presentation). We might be in for a very unpleasant surprise when facing the audience ourselves and, moreover, seeing others perform well in such a situation might even emphasize our own failures.

Public presentations, scary as they might be, are still obviously different from dying and death since the former are not generally bad for us in the way dying and death are. Apart from the fact that we are able to live and tell about the former, dying is also often associated with physically troubling symptoms and the fear related to the occurrences of such symptoms. So, in what way is acquaintance with death supposed to help us to die a better death, and are things different when we compare public presentations and death regarding this? It would seem that possible suggestions are things like finding death and dying less fearful, not being liable to negative surprises to the same extent, being less frustrated in setting realistic goals. It might also result in us knowing better how our desires relate to death and dying or in us *creating* desires in relation to death and dying. This in turn will better enable us to express these desires (to both ourselves and others) when facing dying and death ourselves. Finally, it could be argued that being acquainted with death is instrumentally beneficial in relation to achievements in dying. Lawton (2000) observed how carers at the hospice where she made her study tried to make dying and death public to the other patients, mainly for the benefit of these other patients. Something, she concludes, which is done at the expense of the dying person's need or want for privacy and integrity.

First we have to be aware that facing death and dying will often lower our well-being to some extent, especially if we are in some way emotionally related to the person dying, and it seems strange that we should try to get acquainted with death by attending the death of strangers or people to whom we are only distantly related. Of course, being professionally involved in the care of dying might have its enjoyable moments and on the whole be rewarding. But for those of us not thus involved, facing death and dying involves a cost in well-being. What acquaintance brings us in terms of positive value might of course balance this value loss.

Having this in mind, would I be benefited by earlier experiences of the death and dying of other people when dying myself? We can seldom imagine what it implies (so to say from the inside) that someone else experiences fear or pain or decay or whatever is troubling in dying. For example, I cannot really imagine what it is like to give birth, even having watched my wife give birth to our children. Moreover, I doubt that these experiences would really make it easier for me if I was to face a similar situation. Seeing her give birth actually made me even more grateful that I am a man and do not have to face such an ordeal. That is, seeing other people facing troublesome physical and psychological symptoms does not in any direct way make us more prepared or better at handling these symptoms when they occur in our own lives. Moreover, in relation to the manifold ways we might die it seems that we can still be (negatively) surprised even if acquainted with a number of deaths. Lawton (2000) refers to some studies (Honeybun *et al.* 1992; Payne *et al.* 1996) that claim that patients who witnessed the death of other patients were significantly less depressed. However, her own observations do not support this conclusion, and she relates the goodness of witnessing other patients' deaths to the difficulties these patients face in dying and death. That is, the more gruesome and terrible a death is, the more scared the other patients become about how their own death will be.

Could this be countered by that fact that it would generally be easier to get our desires fulfilled? In encountering a number of deaths from a third person perspective it is likely that we start to think about our own dying and death and how these different dying and death situations accord with our own desires about how we want to be, what we want to do. It might also lead us to formulate new desires or to reconsider our basic desires. Hence it is not unlikely that we, as a result of this, will work out more explicit desires about our own dying and death and have the ability to express them more explicitly when facing our own death.

Suppose I work as a nurse and experience a number of bad deaths where people are kept alive beyond the point where I find life worth living. Then it is not unrealistic that I would form desires about how far I would like to have my life prolonged when facing death myself. (In my own experience, it is not unusual to hear palliative carers say, even given the philosophy of palliative care, which gives precedence to a death from cancer where we have time to prepare for death with most of our mental capacities intact (Walter 1994; Seale 1998), that they would like to die a sudden death in sleep.) Perhaps I might even form desires about wanting death to be induced in order to avoid such an extended death. However, fulfilment does not follow by necessity since the fulfilment of our desires depends on a lot more than having expressed our desires clearly and explicitly to ourselves and others. To continue the example, having worked out in advance that we wish to receive euthanasia when facing a specific type of dying trajectory does not benefit us in relation to the desire fulfilment scale (rather the opposite, in fact), since we are not likely to receive euthanasia even if we desire it ever so much (due to the legal situation in most of the countries of the world).

Moreover, this example indicates that the nature of these desires will depend on what earlier experiences amount to, as Lawton (2000) argues. If we experience a series of 'bad' deaths, we will probably have desires about our own death that are different from those if we experience a series of 'good' deaths. Now it might be argued that such acquaintance will result in us having more realistic desires about dying and death and hence we will fare better when it comes to desire fulfilment. However, to form realistic desires might imply that we lower our expectations to a point that would seem problematic. In Tolstoy's short story 'Master and Man' we meet a rich merchant and his servant who end up in a snowstorm. The merchant struggles to keep alive while Nikita, the servant, 'submits to death patiently and unresistingly . . . This was because he had had few happy feast-days in his life but many bitter weeks, and he was tired of the uninterrupted work' (Tolstoy 1974: 61). Since the servant was familiar with the hardships of life he adapted to the hardship of dying and death without struggle. To me it seems problematic that we could prepare for an easier death by living a life of deprivation in which we have lowered our expectations. In any case, if that would bring us a better death it would be at the cost of a good life.

Following this, prior acquaintance with dying and death will not in any direct way enable us to get more of our desires fulfilled in dying and death. It might even be problematic to the extent that we adapt our desires in a way that will make us lose out on the goods of life. Still, it could be argued that, even if not necessarily beneficial on the hedonistic or desire fulfilment scales of a good life, there might be more objective values that will provide support for prior acquaintance with dying and death. One example would be that we would achieve better in dying and death. However, the parallel with the public presentation did not give us reason to believe so. Moreover, what is problematic with achieving things in the vicinity of death is not necessarily that the things we achieve (if indeed there are such things) are difficult to achieve in themselves but that we have to achieve them in a situation of emotional distress.

For example, if we want to sort out our relational conflicts before we die we might find this difficult, either because we find it difficult to sort out conflicts, so that prior acquaintance with death does not solve anything, or because we find it problematic to do so in the vicinity of death, since that also implies that we are soon to leave these people. If so, it is difficult to see how prior acquaintance with other people's death would actually make conflict-solving easier for us, since that would imply that we could actually learn how to lose someone close without being too emotionally affected. This is something I find difficult to believe we would manage, at least if we want to stay close to people.

In effect, prior acquaintance with dying and death might make us more realistic as to what it implies to sort out conflicts. For example, we might realize that we should not venture to try such an achievement at all. This would obviously spare us a number of possible failures, but on the other hand it would not seem to bring us closer to a good death (if sorting out conflicts is beneficial to such a death) *per se* – only derivatively so if the spared time is put to better use.

Hence the idea that if we face a number of other people's deaths we will thereby be able to achieve well ourselves when we are about to die would not seem very credible except for the fact that it might give us a clue as to what it is we should achieve. On the other hand, this might also be done by reading the kind of literature I am discussing in this book, something that is, I hope, less emotionally distressing. In conclusion, I find rather scarce support for the idea that we generally would be benefited as dying persons by prior acquaintance with dying and death.

Value to others

What about the value to others involved in this situation, i.e. close ones and the carer? It could be argued that there are several aspects to this question. Would the dying person's prior acquaintance benefit close ones and carers? Would close ones' and carers' prior acquaintance benefit the dying person? Would close ones' and carers' prior acquaintance benefit *them*? Following the above discussion, I simply assume that to the extent that the dying person will benefit people in the vicinity of his death by prior acquaintance (which draws on the more general discussion of whether third person acquaintance can benefit from a third person perspective) this might still be compromised by being in the kind of emotionally overwhelming situation he is in.

Now, it might be true that facing a number of deaths from a third person perspective will enable us to face yet other deaths from a third person perspective. For example, in Elias (1985) it is claimed that we might be less at a loss for words when facing dying people if we are already acquainted with dying, which seems plausible to some extent. My own experiences of working with dying people support this and it seems convincing that professional palliative carers who have experience and training in facing dying and death are often better suited than others to care for terminally ill persons. However, at this point it is important to distinguish between close ones and professional carers. As indicated above, there is obviously an emotional cost involved in facing the death of someone close, which is not the case to the same extent when we face the death of a patient when in the role of a professional carer. That is, one important reason why palliative carers can provide good care to the palliative patient is the fact that they are able to strike a balance between distance and closeness in the sense of not getting too emotionally involved in the patient.

On the other hand, the emotional distress faced by close ones might hinder them from putting former experiences with death and dying into practice. Former experiences might of course help us to some extent. If so, we should be acquainted with death in order to help other people die, not to get a better death ourselves. To illustrate, the second time my wife gave birth, my previous experience came in quite handy and I felt less at odds and more able to aid her in her predicament. It might also be argued that previous experience with dying and death will enable us to live a better life. Hence, apart from the fact that we might help others we might also benefit ourselves from such prior acquaintance – though not necessarily when we are dying. This will, however, not be discussed in this context (see Sandman 2001 for a discussion of this).

Normative aspects of an acquainted death

Since prior acquaintance or familiarity with dying and death is not of general value to the dying person he or she will not have any strong reasons to seek out the deaths of other people to prepare for his or her own dying. However, close ones might have some normative reasons to do so in order to benefit the person dying, though we saw that we might not be able to draw effectively on these experiences when we are distressed.

From the perspective of palliative care it is doubtful whether we can actually help dying people to get more aquainted with death and dying in an effective manner. That is a preparation they need to have done before they start to die. Perhaps, if we had found strong support for such acquaintance, palliative care institutions should have offered non-dying people the opportunity to face dying people. However, this would still not have been warranted given the strain and invasion of the privacy of dying people such a practice would have brought. It is also doubtful whether palliative carers should expose other dying patients to dying and death in order to make them more acquainted, especially since they will have to sort out the deaths that actually will bring comfort – a sorting that will emphasize that not all deaths are easy and comforting.

In line with this the best normative strategy of the professional carer is to let patients decide on whether they want to face death and dying before they die or not. Here it is also important to respect the self-determination of those patients who could be the means to such acquaintance: are they willing to act as such means? However, to the extent that all involved parties agree that this is what they want to do, and are aware of the possible risks involved, such as the risk of losing hope or becoming pessimistic about one's own dying, it can be provided.

On the other hand, since the dying person will plausibly benefit from being cared for by people who have prior acquaintance with death and dying there are strong normative reasons for professional carers, caring for dying people, to be experienced in facing the death and dying of others. This will give us reasons to let people die in specific care contexts for dying people where they will face experienced people; or, in order to allow people the opportunity to get good care in different care contexts, to ensure that carers within the full variety of care contexts we might face are experienced in the care of dying people. At the same time, since facing death and dying are supposedly emotionally stressful even for the professional carer, this requires the support of good education and training as well as counselling in order for palliative carers to be able to recover from this emotional strain.

It is, once again, important that the culture of care does not automatically force acquaintance with death and dying upon dying patients who have not explicitly asked for this.

Awareness of death

In the literature on good death the idea that we should be aware of death in the vicinity of death has a strong hold on the palliative community, not least due to the influence of writers like Kübler-Ross, with her stages in dying, and the work on different awareness contexts by Glaser and Strauss (1965). The taxonomy provided by the latter two has been used extensively within the palliative discussion (this is not a full taxonomy since there are several alternatives missing) (Walter 1994; Field 1996; Seale 1998):

- Open awareness: both the dying person and the relatives know that the person is dying.
- Pretence: the dying person or the relative (or both) pretend that they do not know the person is dying.
- Suspicion: the dying person suspects that he or she is dying.
- Closed awareness: the dying person is kept from the knowledge that he or she is dying.

We also find this ideal outside the palliative community. For example, Callahan (1993: 54) claims that a good death should be marked 'by a self-awareness that one is dying, that the end has come'. We also find the idea that we should be aware of death in the midst of life, when not dying; what we might refer to as the idea of *memento mori*. Consider, for example, the following statement by Kübler-Ross (1969: 26): 'I believe that we should make it a habit to think about death and dying occasionally.' However, this will not be dealt with in this context, except in passing (see Sandman 2001 for a more thorough discussion on this).

Generally, awareness of death seems to imply that *I*, in one sense, have accepted that *I* am going to die. That is, I have cognitively accepted that I am about to die, which does not necessarily imply that I have accepted death in other senses of the term. Elaborating somewhat on the idea of acceptance of death, it would seem that acceptance can mean at least three (possibly four) different things when applied to a good death.

First, we can accept death in terms of having a cognitive attitude to death, where the opposite attitude is denial. In Kübler-Ross (1969) denial is one of the earlier stages to go through before we reach the stage of acceptance. To accept death cognitively is then to believe some fact about death to be true or justified or applicable in this situation. We accept the fact that we humans are mortal, or accept the fact that *I* am mortal, or accept that death is closing in on *me*.

Second, we can accept death in terms of having an emotional attitude to death, where the opposite attitude is defiance. That is, we relate in specific ways to the approaching (or possibly approaching) death (which, in most cases, seem to presuppose cognitive acceptance of death). To accept death emotionally is to let go of life, not to fight against death, to welcome death, to surrender in front of death.[3] This is dealt with in the next section, on acceptance of death.

Third, we can accept death in terms of evaluating death as something good or at least neutral or acceptable (in this situation or generally). Not to accept death in these terms would imply evaluating it as something bad or evil (in this situation or generally). However, since I find this to be of more peripheral interest it is dealt with only in passing in the next section.

Fourth, we can bodily accept death, implying that our body seems to let the disease have its way, without using any of its defence mechanisms.[4] When the best timing of death has arrived, it could be claimed that bodily acceptance would be in our best interest and, hence, conducive to a good death. If, on the other hand, the best timing of death has not arrived, bodily acceptance would not be in our best interest. However, it seems that this is the only way bodily acceptance might be relevant to a good death so it is ignored in the following. Moreover, it seems that we might have greater difficulty in influencing whether our physiological organism accepts death or not.

As indicated above, we might cognitively accept death in a number of different ways and this acceptance might take on different faces: we might cognitively accept that man is mortal, we might cognitively accept that we are mortal and, following Ivan Illych in Tolstoy's short story about Ivan's death, we might accept the former but not the latter: ' "Caius is a man; men are mortal; therefore Caius is mortal" had always seemed to him correct as applied to Caius, but certainly not as applied to himself' (Tolstoy 1974). We might also cognitively accept that we are going to die soon (i.e. that we are dying in line with the way 'dying' is used in this book). Now, cognitive acceptance would seem to be of little importance unless it results in awareness of the fact that we are dying or the fact that we are mortal. That is, if we could cognitively accept death and then suffer partial amnesia, cognitive acceptance would seem neither good nor bad for us; or if we could block out the awareness after having received information, what Field and Copp (1999: 465) call 'suspended awareness'. Hence, below I focus on the awareness of death that cognitive acceptance results in.

Value to the dying person and others

To accept cognitively that we are dying implies becoming aware of or allowing one to become aware of the fact that the remaining time in life is short. This awareness might be had in degrees (for example, constantly being aware of this) or intermittently (for example, actualized when making important decisions), or just having it as a background attitude.[5] In Field and Copp (1999) these latter versions are referred to as conditional openness (see Glaser and Strauss's taxonomy above). As Field and Copp suggest, this might be a way out of the extremes, i.e open awareness or denial. However, in this context I will focus on these more extreme attitudes, especially since the fully open awareness attitude is the one advocated in palliative philosophy to a large extent (Walter 1994).

In this context I will take a look at three different types of arguments for awareness or against denial being conducive to a good death. If we are meticulous, not being aware and denying do not amount to exactly the same things. The latter seems to presuppose that we have or get some information, but deny it to be true, while in the former case the lack of awareness might actually depend on lack of information. However, in this context I will treat them as mutually exclusive of each other. Now, it might be impossible to remain unaware of the fact that we are dying in many cases. However, not being successful in denying oncoming death does not imply anything concerning the goodness or badness of such denial. That is, the world is unfortunately not so wisely created as to make everything that is good for us easily available; on the contrary, what is good might often seem difficult to achieve. Moreover, as is argued in, for example, Field (1996) and Seale (1998), to interpret the signals that we are dying might be easier given a certain kind of diagnosis, e.g. cancer and AIDS, but more difficult in relation to other types of diagnoses that are no less fatal, e.g. cardiovascular problems.

Here are the arguments. First, awareness is instrumentally useful, in that it will enable us to take advantage of the time we have left – for example, care for our close ones, prepare for death in different ways, take evasive actions against death or just focus on the things that will bring value to the time we have left. Second, awareness will be conducive to self-determination, freedom and control over one's life. Third, awareness is valuable in itself, being an essential part of a good life.

Richard W. Momeyer (1998: 4–5) in his *Confronting Death* claims that:

> Indeed, [denial] might hasten death's arrival by occasioning the failure to take effective evasive action. Not being prepared for departure means a difficult exit, one the usually leaves much unfinished business behind . . . Denial, by inviting pretense and hypocrisy from all who attempt communication with the dying, taints precisely those relations it is intended to protect . . . denial ill prepares one for dying.

Peter Noll, a Swiss Professor of Law, claims in his *Diktate über Sterben und Tod mit Totenrede von Max Frisch*:

> You will choose with greater consideration among the innumerable possibilities in life and no longer just accept those that conventionally lead to a fast career or, if you already have a high position, not collect one position after another just to be on the very top. This is the wasted, lost time, not that spent together with a woman or in conversation

with friends. On the other hand you will postpone fewer tasks to the future . . . you will ask: What have I neglected? What should I spend more time on? What would give more meaning? Which moments have I not used sufficiently, which should be used more? . . . Show those who care for you more love, devote less attention to those who do not care for you.

(Noll 1985: 76, 77 my translation)

Awareness in these quotations is supposed to result in bringing us a better life in the time that is left in one of three ways: in buying us more time, in preparing us for the end or in enabling us to use the time we have left in a better way.

Let us start with the possibility of buying more time. If a woman denies or ignores or is unaware of the lump in her chest being cancer she will most probably fail to get a mastectomy and instead of having a chance of surviving (at least for some time) she will possibly die. To the extent that further life would have been good for her it seems obvious that she made a loss in not being thus aware.

However, as indicated in the above comments on different diagnoses and their being ' "scripted into" the discourse on aware dying' (Seale *et al.* 1997: 478), we often get treatment for otherwise fatal conditions without having to acknowledge that we are actually dying. That is, if we are suffering from a fatal disease, we cannot deny this to the point of not even contacting a doctor or the hospital. But it seems possible, even if not easily so, to acknowledge that we are in pain or suffering and ask the doctor to do something about these symptoms or generally to admit to the doctor that we are willing do everything to get well or to live as long as possible and still deny that we are actually dying.[6]

Moreover, when we are in a condition where nothing can be done to cure our condition and only marginal survival is an option, what can be done might be of less value to us and hence will have to be weighed against the obvious suffering that would seem to result from being aware of the fact that we are dying. In Maguire and Faulkner's words: 'Patients use denial when the truth is too painful to bear. So denial should not be challenged unless it is creating serious problems for the patient or relative' (Maguire and Faulkner 1993: 190). This would also seem to be supported in Lawton (2000), where talk about the future (which obviously involves death) is interpreted as taboo and where patients do not seem to want to be reminded of the fact that they are soon to be dead, even if they are aware of this in some sense (see also Field and Copp 1999).

What about Momeyer's other suggestion, that in denying death we will not have time to make the preparations needed? In Seale *et al.*'s words:

Relatives can be called to the sick bed, practical and emotional affairs can be set in order, loss can be anticipated and grieving begun by both

dying people and those close to them. Plans can be made for the negotiation of a dying career, involving choices of care and the place of
death.

(Seale *et al*. 1997: 477)

The success of this argument rests on the claim that these preparations are
essential to achieve a good death. In other words, making these preparations
will bring value to our dying. This is to some extent dealt with in the
chapters to follow. However, to anticipate that discussion somewhat, there it
will be concluded that the benefits of these preparations would be of varying
value to the dying person and in many cases we would instead have a moral
reason to do them. That is, we should do them because they will benefit
other people. For example, some studies do suggest that if close ones have
the chance to start preparing, emotionally, for the passing away of their
loved one they will have an easier mourning period after the dying person is
dead (Swarte *et al*. 2003). If so, we would have a moral reason to accept and
be aware of oncoming death in order to do what is morally required of us.
On the other hand, since it might be difficult to affect the timing of our own
death, we have reasons to do some of the things we have moral reasons to do
before we die long before we are dying in order to safeguard these benefits.
This concerns primarily setting one's emotional and practical affairs in
order; it is obviously difficult to help people to start to grieve or anticipate
the loss of me long before I am actually dying without affecting the ongoing
relationship for the worse.

Next, Noll's argument is that awareness will make time more valuable to
us and hence make it more important what we do with our time. The general
idea here is that the marginal utility of time increases as the amount of time
decreases. Hence, the less time we have at our disposal, the more important
it is what we do with it if we want our lives to be as valuable as possible. This
seems like a reasonable idea.

In effect, when we have a short time in life left it will be important to be
aware of this in order not to waste time on things that do not add any (or
add little) value to our lives. For example, in Edgar (1996a: 40) it is claimed,
referring to a study on terminally ill cancer patients, that: 'faced with a finite
future, patients reassessed the priorities in their lives, so that long-term and
abstract objectives were replaced by short-term and concrete goals, such as
the enjoyment of family life.' A few points need to be mentioned here. First,
we might live the kind of life where we find constant well-being and desire
fulfilment in what we do every day (even when we strive for long-term and
abstract objectives) and hence we cannot really change it in a way that will
bring us more value, especially given the cost of awareness. Second, if we do
not live on the whole good lives, to what extent can we actually change our
lives in a way that will add value, just by making priorities? That is, would
such changes be of more than marginal value? Third, if dying is a result of

terminal disease we might find ourselves weakened by disease to the point of having to make priorities anyway, without actually admitting to the fact that we are dying (Lawton 2000). Fourth, awareness of oncoming death might make us lose interest in valuable things or things that will add to our lives, questioning the point of doing them when we are about to die.[7] In Glaser and Strauss (1965: 103) it has been argued that the aware patient may die with less dignity (in the aristocratic sense) than if she were unaware of her terminality. In effect, awareness might not only make her lose interest in what adds to her life but also make it difficult for her to be the way she wants to be.

Here we might bring in another aspect of this, that even if we are aware of our own oncoming death we might not be interested in sharing this with other people, since they will start to treat us in a way that will make our lives be over, long before we are actually physically dead. In Lawton (2000: 49–50) we find a woman whose fear of this is actually realized:

> Whilst Fiona was aware of the serious nature of her cancer, she had chosen not to 'dwell on it' or to discuss her prognosis in depth with her family, because she wanted her life to remain 'normal for as long as possible'.
>
> Fiona's anxieties appeared to be well founded. Once her husband had finished his research [into the nature and prognosis of Fiona's condition], his behaviours altered markedly towards her. He changed their disabled daughter's attendance allowance into his own name without consulting her. When he did finally inform Fiona of his actions, he explained that he had to prepare for the future, a future in which she would be gone. Fiona complained that her husband had started treating her as if she were 'already dead'.
>
> (Lawton 2000: 49–50)

Here the shared awareness results in problems for Fiona continuing to live normally 'for as long as possible', even if we might claim that she has a moral reason to make preparations of this kind, if it would cause serious trouble not doing them before she died. However, often it seems that these kinds of preparations could be made after the person is dead, without any real inconvenience to the remaining close ones.

Now, even if we accept the reason for being aware in dying, it seems important not to make a virtue out of necessity, i.e. claim that the period of dying is better than the rest of life because it results in using time more effectively in adding what is valuable to our lives. When we are discussing the more general version of acceptance and awareness of death, the idea that we should be aware of and prepared that death might come at any moment, it could be argued that some of the valuable things in life actually imply that we believe we have considerable time at our disposal to make us motivated to engage in them. Constantly asking questions like 'Am I doing the most valuable thing, given the circumstances? Am I using my time optimally?' would seem distressful and the suspicion that we are actually wasting our time might gnaw away at us. Consequently, in order to live a good life, we need to take time off from the conscious search for a good life, to relax, dare to try out things even if they turn out wrong, waste time. John Harris seems to have a point in claiming that if 'life had a short and finite (rather than indefinite) future, most things would not seem worth doing' (Harris 1985: 100; see also Seale 1998).

The other part of Noll's argument relates to the impact on relationships awareness of imminent death will have: 'Show those who care for you more love, devote less attention to those who do not care for you. Become more patient where you used to be impatient, calmer where you once were worried, more open and harder where you were lenient and opportunistic' (Noll 1985: 77, my translation). Would awareness that time is scarce lead to such a change in our relationships and, if so, would such a change be beneficial to us? More generally, how will awareness versus denial affect our relationships, and will it affect them in a way that will make a difference to the way they add to our lives?

The important implication of the quotation is that we should spend our limited time with the people we have intimate personal relationships with instead of the people who are only instrumentally valuable to us. That is, when we have ample time at our disposal (or believe we have ample time at our disposal), we need to spend time and effort on people with whom we have no intimate personal relationships, since they are instrumental in bringing value in different ways to our lives. When things change and we only have a small amount of time left in life, we will probably not have enough time to realize the value resulting from such instrumental relationships or the intimate personal relationships will bring us more value. If so, awareness of imminent death will give us the opportunity to change priorities during the limited time left in life.

However, first we are obviously often instrumentally dependent on other people even when we are imminently dying; for example, professional carers. Second, since we might be aware of oncoming death for quite some time we might have to continue working or we might have time to make important achievements for which other people will be instrumental. Moreover, we need to remember that on any of the value approaches, close relationships are not all there is to a good life. Hence, we can have reasons to make other priorities when we have limited time at our disposal, and perhaps the combination of things we normally fill our lives with and continue to fill our lives with (given limited energy due to disease) is the best combination there is. That is to say, if we give all of our time to our close ones we might actually lose out on other valuables.

Even if we concentrate on close relationships, it is not obvious that open awareness of death and dying will always be beneficial. According to

Weisman (1972: 63) mutual denial might even be beneficial to the relationship in not causing it unnecessary strain (see also Field and Copp 1999). On the other hand, being aware might enable close ones to be open about what will happen and then affirm a 'secure social bond' (Seale 1998: 175) and care for the dying person, and also to be present when the person dies (Seale *et al.* 1997). However, others report that denial or less than full awareness will make them better suited to care for their loved one and to continue as normal, and will not cause them to despair (Seale 1998). Walter (1994) highlights that patients may deny oncoming death in order to spare close ones and care personnel. Moreover, many authors report differences in how awareness is viewed in different cultures (see, for example, Seale *et al.* 1997; Field and Copp 1999 for references), where closed awareness or denial on behalf of the patient is the norm, and not something that will cause problems to the relationships; on the contrary, their awareness is viewed as something that will cause damage to the dying person and the relationship. Hence, the relationship might be preserved or benefited in different ways, depending on the relationship and on the parties to the relationship. This might to some extent be dependent on different views on close relationships. In Walter (1994) it is argued that the open awareness attitude is in line with an expressivism concerning emotions that also reflects on what a healthy close relationship amounts to. In line with the above, we can always question whether this is the only way we can have close relationships with each other. However, as Lawton (2000) points out, it might be problematic when the parties in a relationship take on different attitudes to awareness of death. Hence, it would generally seem to be of benefit if they agree on how to deal with awareness of dying and death.

The second type of argument relates to the complex we might call autonomy (i.e. things like self-determination, freedom and control or independence; see Sandman 2004 for a further analysis of autonomy). In the discussion of awareness in dying, it has been argued that this is closely related to the kind of modern individualism in which control over the trajectory of one's life and making one's life into one's own project is central (see, for example, Walter 1994; Field 1996; Seale 1998). Here we will take a look at some ideas suggesting that awareness is beneficial in relation to self-determination, freedom and control.

We start with the claim that awareness of death will make us freer in relation to life. Consider the following statement from Noll: 'No one can take away more than life from us, and this will anyhow be taken away' (Noll 1985: 103, my translation). One interpretation of what Noll says is that the worst deprivation we can suffer is the deprivation of life and, if we are soon to die, we will soon be deprived of life and nothing really matters in comparison to that. Consequently, we might act more freely (i.e. have more alternatives we actually can choose), since any deprivation we might suffer as a result of acting thus will be relatively small in comparison.

Another interpretation is that after we have been deprived of life, we cannot be deprived of anything more. With this interpretation, we might be freer near the end of life, since, once dead, we will not have to suffer the consequences of what we did when alive, and even if we do not miss out on these consequences altogether we will not suffer them for long.

Let us start with the first half of the first interpretation. In Chapter 3, when discussing the badness of death, it was concluded that the most important factor for why death is bad for us is the deprivation factor and, according to this factor, we can suffer worse deprivations than being deprived of life. This implies that death is sometimes the least bad alternative for us. For example, if the victim of torture dies when under torture, he would seem to have gotten the better deal of the deals available, and the torturers might be annoyed with him getting away. That is, for a victim of torture it would seem rational to fear the suffering of torture more than the loss of his life.

Hence, if we risked torture as a result of acting freely even if we were about to die, this would not seem to motivate us to become more free. That is to say, it is not irrational to find torture worse than death and, if so, knowing that we are about to die will not necessarily make us freer. On the other hand, if death is actually the result of acting more freely, would awareness that we are soon to die make a difference as to how we would act in relation to such an option? That is, does it matter to us if we die a week earlier than we would have died if we had not acted as freely? Following the previous discussion about the marginal utility of small measures of time, it would not seem indifferent to us if we die a week earlier. Interestingly enough, here we seem to find a conflict between the first person perspective of having a week left in life and the overall perspective on life. That is, from the overall perspective it would not seem to make much difference whether I am deprived of an extra week or not (even if it makes some difference). However, from the first person perspective, knowing that we only have a week left would seem to make that week very valuable indeed and we might not be willing to lose it. Hence, from the overall perspective we could become daredevils at the end of our lives but from the first person perspective we are likely to remain cautious.

Even admitting to this we might agree with Noll that there are few things that actually are worse than being deprived of life. If the result of what we could do were not torture or death or something of sorts, would awareness that we are about to die make us freer? First, the way we act in different situations might be the result of deep-rooted character traits, not easily changed just because we are aware of limited time left in life. Second, if death is not a result of any choice we would have in the situation, would it really make much difference to what we do to compare the alternative outcomes with death? If someone told me that speaking my mind to the boss cannot be worse than death, I would probably say 'so what?' and continue to be as reluctant to do this as before. That is, we do not seem to be psychologically constructed in a way that would make such comparisons actually work in making us freer. If anything, it is becoming convinced that the situation *per se* is not as bad as we imagine that can make us freer, not that there are worse things that can happen to us, especially not when these worse things are not actually options in the situation. I do not see any reasons why things would be generally different if we are soon to die. In conclusion, I do not find the idea that we would be freer if we compare the outcomes of our alternatives with the outcome of death convincing.

What about the second interpretation? This implies that since death will release us from the consequences of what we do (or, at least, the long-term consequences) we might be less afraid of doing what we want. Moreover, we might find a stronger motivation to do things we are afraid of because of the belief that we will have few opportunities left to do them. I find this a plausible idea. If I knew that after having spoken my mind to the boss I would drop dead, I would feel freer to do or say whatever I wanted to and perhaps even be able to suppress my terror of doing this. (I must admit, though, that if I had only a couple of hours at my disposal before dying, I would not opt for speaking my mind to the boss.) To take a less drastic example, I think we generally find it easier to speak our mind to people at work if we are about to leave for another job at another place, since we do not have to suffer the consequences of being frank and outspoken to a great extent. That is, awareness of imminent death might make us less afraid of speaking our mind. The reason for this is that what are at stake are things like suffering a bad reputation, being ignored and being hindered from achieving good things in the future, and when there is little time left we will not have much time to experience these consequences of our actions.

To the extent that the things we could do as a result of such awareness are beneficial to us, it will be instrumentally good to be aware of oncoming death. On the other hand, this might not be an unmitigated good (at least not to others), since it might also make us commit immoral actions or actions hurtful to others, believing that we will never have to suffer the consequences.

In conclusion, I find it plausible that we will become somewhat freer in relation to actions with problematic consequences as a result of knowing that we do not have to suffer the consequences of these actions, and this will add to our lives to the extent that we use this freedom to do things that are valuable on any of the value accounts. Still, it remains to be shown that these benefits outweigh the obvious cost of accepting and being aware of imminent death. In other words, are there really a lot of things we abstain from doing because we do not want to suffer the consequences, things we can do at the end of life and that would actually benefit us? I am doubtful! Moreover, some of these things might normally be associated with bad consequences (i.e. other people's sanctions) because they are hurtful to other people.

Moving on to self-determination and control or independence, could the value of deciding the destiny of one's life and controlling the extent to which those decisions are implemented support being aware of death at the end of life? Given the formulation of self-determination in Chapter 2, it would seem that the person who denies oncoming death and thereby hands over control over his life to someone else might also be considered to be self-determined as long as this is the result of a decision that is in line with his wants. This is so if the decision (to the extent that it is a decision) to deny and not involve himself in the decision-making is not forced on him or something he is manipulated into doing or has done under the influence of drugs. That is, if it is a consequence of who he is and what he believes and values, the denial would seem autonomous. Now, it might be argued that in being under duress he is in fact forced into taking such a decision and it is not *his* decision or a decision he would take when not under duress. I find this a difficult claim to evaluate. First, even if it has some initial plausibility, it seems doubtful that we should judge this as a situation of force. Obviously, there is not another person forcing me, if anything it is the circumstances (external as well as internal) that 'force' me to deny death. If we allow the circumstances, i.e. the state of the external world and the state of my character and personality, to be potential forces in relation to self-determination, we would never be self-determined since we would always be more or less (often more) influenced by these circumstances. To illustrate, surely my decision to run when facing a couple of hoodlums is a self-determined decision even if it is the result of the external circumstance (being threatened) and my personality (being a coward). That is, given who I am this is what I actually want to do in that situation. Consequently, I think we will have to interpret the situation of denial as a situation where the person is actually acting and deciding self-determinedly on a reasonable account of what self-determination amounts to. On the other hand, if it is important for the dying person to participate in every decision about his remaining life, whether it concerns treatment or whatever, awareness will of course be necessary, as Lawton (2000) notes.

When it concerns control or independence (i.e. the ability to influence the outcome of our decisions and perform the actions we want to perform) it would seem that awareness is beneficial, since in accepting that we are going to die, we might arrange our final days in the way we want (given the circumstances). However, we might also interpret the denying person as exercising control over his dying, i.e. in denying he might control what is valuable to him, which are not things like influencing the exact place or time of death (see Seale 1998). That is, they might not be interested in entering what Field (1996) has called the modern dying role but want to fashion another role for themselves or remain in the role they have had through the rest of life. In other words, what the denying person might view as important to control are things like not being overwhelmed by suffering, not losing the motivation to continue to live life as normally as possible or not losing dignity (according to the above). This might also be something that is related to a certain self-identity where I struggle to take control over the threatening influence of the external world in whatever way possible. Hence, from the perspective of controlling what life I live, or what person I am, it is not obvious that awareness is necessarily the best attitude to adopt. It all depends on what I want to control or what kind of control is necessary in order to live the life I want to live or a life in line with who I am. Seale *et al.* (1997) have noticed a certain relation to class in what awareness attitude one adopts, where the educated, home-owning class was more prone to be aware of death and dying. This is thought to underline the connection between awareness and individualistic control, since the higher classes are supposed to be more influenced by this modern project. However, it could also be that these different classes have different individualistic projects going on, i.e. more related to what kind of self-identity and role is important and what means to use to achieve this, rather than about adopting or not adopting the project of fashioning life for oneself as best possible.

On the other hand, whether or not one is aware might not be the result of a conscious decision and hence not a result of self-determination but a consequence of being a certain person or living under certain circumstances, or even the result of someone else's decision. Still, when it is not the result of someone else's decision, it might still be the result of whom I have chosen to become and in line with my self-identity. However, Field and Copp (1999) report a study where the findings seem to show that patients are able to control their level of awareness in a way that is tolerable to them.

How would the dying person's denial or awareness affect the freedom and self-determination of other people? Given what we mean by self-determination they will still be able to make their own decisions, even if the alternatives might have changed. That is, they will still be self-determined but their freedom has changed, even if it is an open question whether it is lessened or not. When it comes to control over their lives, it will once again depend on what they find important to control. The example from Lawton (2000) above, where the husband of a dying patient, Fiona, arranged for the future lives of him and their handicapped daughter, shows that from his perspective he found awareness essential to be able to control what would happen when Fiona died. Hence, once again, it might be problematic when we have different ideas on what it is essential to control, or what is essential in order to fashion a good life for oneself. However, as suggested above, in the Western world we often live under circumstances where postponing the planning of our future lives will not cause any serious inconvenience to us. That is, the welfare system might be able to cover us for the period it takes to arrange our lives according to the changed situation. If not, the dying person might have a moral reason to become aware to the extent that this will markedly enable close ones to have an easier future.

What about Momeyer's other argument in favour of cognitive acceptance and awareness? Consider the following claim:

> what death denial requires is that we not face and acknowledge the meaner realities of living, not just with respect to death and dying, but in all of our relationships and experiences. Denial and avoidance of unpleasantness – where dying is an ultimate unpleasantness – make for a superficial life, one perhaps conventionally respectable but finally hollow . . . [denial] fails as a satisfying way of living.
>
> (Momeyer 1988: 5)

Here Momeyer advocates an idea about facing up to life or being in contact with reality whatever it will bring along, claiming that what he calls 'the unexamined life . . . [is] not worth living' (*ibid.*). Starting with the well-being approach, only what enters our mind can affect the value of our lives, and being deprived of bad experiences is better than not being thus deprived. Hence, such an approach would actually claim that we should avoid the 'meaner realities' of this world unless we thereby lose out on some greater good.

What about the desire fulfilment approach: what does that imply for the idea about facing up to realities as essential for a worthwhile life? Well, a desire of ours could obviously be fulfilled even if we do not know about it. For example, if we desire not to be slandered it would be bad for us to be slandered even if we never get to know about it. However, we might have a desire not to be slandered but also a desire not to know about it if we are. In such a case it would still be as bad for us to be slandered but better if we do not get to know about it when we are.

Likewise, in relation to dying and death, in not accepting or being aware of soon approaching death we will not avoid the badness of what we avert in dying and death, the ending of our lives. On the other hand, getting to know about it does not add anything good to our lives, especially not if we desire to remain in ignorance about these things. Hence, from a desire fulfilment approach, facing up to reality has no intrinsic value and how it will add to a life depends on what desires we have about it. If we deny our oncoming death it seems likely that the reason we do so is because we actually desire to remain in ignorance about this. At this point we need to remember, however, that in not acknowledging what is happening we might not be able to fulfil other relevant desires, such as saying goodbye to close ones or finally doing what we have postponed for so long. Still, the value of fulfilling these desires will, obviously, have to be weighed against the negative value associated with getting to know about oncoming death.

Consequently, it seems the best support for Momeyer's idea would be found in the objective list approach, more specifically in the idea of reality contact. Is it finally good for us to be in contact with reality or is it generally instrumentally good for us to be in contact with reality? Starting with the latter question there are obviously cases where it would be instrumentally detrimental if we knew the full truth about the situation.

Consider the following (true) story.[8] A Swedish surgeon was for a number of years the most skilled surgeon in Scandinavia at performing a certain operation. As it happened his own daughter was taken ill in a way that required this operation and the surgeon was faced with the decision whether he, the most skilled surgeon, should perform the operation or leave it to someone else less skilled. He realized, since the operation required full concentration, that if he knew he was operating on his daughter he would probably be so concerned with what would happen if he failed that it would affect his performance for the worse. As it turned out, he operated on his daughter but was unaware of the fact that it was his daughter. He said afterwards: 'Had I realized during the operation that it was my daughter I was operating on, I could not have gone through with the operation.' Here we have a case where reality contact would be detrimental to the good of the situation.

We might find an abundance of examples like this one, where the full knowledge of the situation would seem to impair us in aquiring some good. However, we might accept these situations and still claim that if it had not been detrimental to our venture we would have been better off knowing the full truth about the situation (perhaps claiming that it would have made it into an even greater achievement). In other words, reality contact is finally good but might be instrumentally bad in some situations and all things equal it is better to be in contact with reality than not.

Let us take another example. A group of people living at some distance from where I live have heard about my opinions on good death and have as a result of that started to dislike or even hate me. Now, some people would claim that in an objective list account it is bad for us if people hate us even if we never get to know about it and even if it does not have any instrumentally bad effects on our lives. Someone arguing from contact with reality would claim that we are actually better off if we get to know about people hating us. To me, even accepting the first idea, the second one seems blatantly wrong. Even if it is bad for us if people, unknowingly to us, hate us at a distance it would certainly not seem better for us to get to know about it.

Ignoring the suffering such knowledge might give rise to (since we have assumed that such knowledge does not have any instrumentally bad effects on our lives), I cannot see any reasons why our lives would be better off knowing about this hate. Hence, even if we find some credibility in the idea about reality contact, it would seem that we might find it reasonable to put a restriction on this idea, with the effect that reality contact is only finally good for us to the extent that it implies being in contact with a reality that is beneficial to us (even if it might often be instrumentally good for us to be in contact even with the meaner realities of life). In relation to dying and death such a restriction would be relevant, since it has been argued that dying and death are generally bad for us.

Hence, I have some difficulties accepting the idea about reality contact, since it has some problematic implications. If we accept it, I find it relevant to put a restriction on the idea in terms of it only being beneficial to be in contact with the reality that is beneficial to us, unless it is of instrumental use to be in such a contact. Still, it might sometimes be of instrumental use to other people that we are thus aware. Hence, we might on occasion have moral reasons to be aware of reality, even the meaner aspects of this reality.

Summary

In conclusion, it can be said that we find reasons supporting both awareness and denial in the face of death and dying, but they cannot be said to support conclusively either awareness or denial. That awareness is necessary to take steps and measures for avoiding otherwise premature death was questioned, since that involves awareness not necessarily that we are dying, just that we are ill. That awareness is necessary to make certain preparations is of course true. However, the strength of this argument will depend on whether these preparations are important enough to warrant the problematic awareness of oncoming death and also whether they actually do presuppose awareness of death in the vicinity of death. That awareness of death might make the time left more valuable was found to have some support, but once again the strength of this argument depends on whether the priorities we make as a result of this would not be done anyway and whether they actually bring that much more value to our lives. That awareness would be beneficial to our relationships was found to have ambigious support, even if it seems reasonable that a joint attitude, whether awareness or denial, would be the best. That awareness might somewhat enhance our freedom to do things at the end of life was found to have some support, but it is not certain that this newly won freedom would be morally acceptable. That awareness is necessarily beneficial to self-determination is not evident: it will depend on what our actual values and desires are. Likewise, when it comes to control, it will depend on what we need to control in our lives. Finally, that awareness would be of final value was not found to have any strong support.

Hence, whether awareness is beneficial to a good death will to a large extent depend on what we find important in life and what we need to control, whether it is important that we are able to continue to live the kind of life we have lived and maintain hope, or to fashion the last days in a specific manner. If we try to find a stronger reason for awareness than what fits best with our own way to live life, we might have moral reasons to become aware of oncoming death when not doing so will cause our close ones serious trouble.

Normative aspects of an aware death

Following the above discussion and the ambivalence in relation to awareness of death, we can make only a few general comments. First, if we accept the idea that we should be extremely careful in overriding the self-determination of the competent patient, we have strong reasons to accept the denial of a patient, even in cases where we judge this denial to be detrimental to him in different ways. An obvious problem here is that in other cases we can try to present the alternatives as vividly as possible, which is not possible here without taking him out of denial or unawareness. However, it seems we can still go a long way towards enabling the patient to decide on treatments and measures to ease his situation or prolong his life without actually bringing him out of denial.

If the denial or unawareness of the patient causes problems for the professional carer in having to be careful with what they say or express, it would seem that this is not a strong enough reason to bring the patient out of denial. This should be part of the role as professional carer and solved by professional support.

On the other hand, if the patient's denial risks the long-term well-being of close ones and the best evidence sees no possibilities of aiding the close ones with these problems after the patient is dead, it would seem that the professional carer has a strong reason to try to bring the patient to the point where he can do what the close ones require, if possible without bringing him out of denial, but if the consequences are serious enough, even to the point of making him aware of oncoming death.

The situation is not symmetric when it comes to denying close ones, since they will eventually face awareness of the patient's death. Hence, even if the consequences of the close ones' denial are less severe for the patient (at least given the shorter perspective) they might still be serious enough for the close ones to have a moral reason to be aware of the oncoming death of the patient. Hence, the professional carer has reasons to try to make close ones aware of the fact that the patient is dying, even if this is to disrespect somewhat the self-determination of the close ones. However, this would seem less problematic, since it is only a matter of a short time until the close ones will have to become aware of the patient's death. Here it is important for the professional carer to try to be clear over why the close ones deny the oncoming death of the patient and how awareness would correspond to the close ones' more fundamental values and ideas.

If a close-one chooses to deny (or ignore) the oncoming death of the dying person even when the professional carer has made it very clear what can be expected for the future, it must obviously be accepted. The reason why self-determination could be somewhat overruled in this case is that the exercise of self-determination is likely to hurt someone else seriously. Important here is that we do not take a specific view on the best attitude to adopt, i.e. awareness or not, as part of the care culture, and influence patients and their close ones in a certain direction without looking at the individual case at hand.

Acceptance of death

In the above section we dealt with cognitive acceptance and awareness of death. In this section we deal with what was called emotional acceptance above. Emotional acceptance involves having an emotional attitude to death, where the opposing attitude might be termed defiance. In the above it was claimed that to accept death emotionally amounts to a range of different attitudes like letting go of life, not fighting against death, welcoming death, surrendering in front of death. It is interesting to note that the attitude of awareness and emotional acceptance, which within the palliative context are considered to move alongside one another, here might part if one of the reasons for awareness is to gain control over dying and death and not surrender to what is coming.

This is, among a number of authors, viewed as central to a good death. Avery D. Weisman claims that an appropriate death implies that 'The patient both accepts and expects death, and is willing, albeit ruefully, to die' (Weisman 1973: 370). Daniel Callahan (1993: 54) says: '[In order to arrive at a peaceful death we need] to fashion a notion of the self that has, in some sustaining way, come to accept death, a self that understands that control over fate will pass from its hands, that this is precisely what biological death means and must mean.' In Kübler-Ross (1969: 100) we find the following statement: '[Acceptance] is as if the pain had gone, the struggle is over and there comes a time for "the final rest before the long journey"'. In Kübler-Ross (1969, 1974), acceptance is the final stage we reach in dying (or at least should reach if we have moved through all the different stages).[9] Following this, emotional acceptance seems to have a strong standing as something that makes for a good dying.

This attitude can be attained by degrees, i.e. we can joyfully or restfully welcome death or just accept it reluctantly, listlessly or ruefully (as is indicated in the above comments from Weisman and Kübler-Ross). Lawton (2000: 79–80) reports that the dying patients in her study do not seem to reach 'a peaceful state of acceptance . . . The overwhelming impression I gained from patients was that their feelings were those of dulled resignation; of apathy, lethargy and exhaustion; of finally giving up.' Moreover, as Lawton notes, this would seem to be related not to their oncoming death *per se*, but to the fact that their bodily (and mental) decay makes it impossible for them to act in a more defying way, even if they want to.

It seems reasonable to assume that the emotional and the cognitive attitude will often move hand in hand even if they are logically independent of each other. That is, if we try to deny death cognitively it is unlikely that we will then emotionally accept it even if the contrary is not true, i.e. that we have to accept death emotionally when we cognitively accept it. Consider the following statement: 'the harder they struggle to avoid the inevitable death, the more they try to deny it' (Kübler-Ross 1969: 101). Even having cognitively accepted death we might still adopt a number of different attitudes to death, ranging from emotional acceptance to emotional defiance. Some claim that even if we accept death cognitively we will always have a hard time accepting it emotionally.[10] If emotional acceptance, on the one hand, implies coming to terms with the situation, adjusting to the situation and not fighting it, expressed, for example, in the Christian martyrs and their joyful anticipation of death[11] but also recommended for 'ordinary' dying people,[12] defiance, on the other hand, implies a conflict between us and the situation, well formulated in the poem by Dylan Thomas (1952):[13]

Do not go gentle into that good night,
Old age should burn and rave at the close of day;
Rage, rage against the dying of the light.

. . .

And you, my father, there on the sad height,
Curse, bless me now with your fierce tears, I pray.
Do not go gentle into that good night.
Rage, rage against the dying of the light.

Value to the dying person and others

As the poem expresses, defiance normally involves struggle and emotional turbulence – anger, aggravation – but also states like endurance paired with loss of hope. From a well-being perspective, emotional acceptance would, on the whole, seem to be a state of experiential well-being; while defiance is more equivocal. That is, the states involved in defiance might both raise and lower the well-being of the person and what dominates is, at least partly, decided by what is achieved by defiance. It is probably satisfying when my defiance leads to some change of the situation and it is more problematic to defy in vain. In Widgery (1993: 19) it is claimed that 'to die fighting death is to cause yourself intractable pain . . . Yet other people can derive an almost exhilarating sense of purpose from the same situation.' Hence, on the face of it, especially since to defy death probably does not lead to any significant change, emotional acceptance would seem to be the best well-being strategy, at least if it is a more positive acceptance (Ågren 1992, 1995); something that Lawton in the quotation above scarcely found among the dying patients she studied.

However, if defiance results in a prolongation of life that is on the whole good and worth the cost of defiance, and emotional acceptance will lead to a shortening of life worth living, defiance would be the best strategy. Hence, adopting the following idea about emotional acceptance, referred to in Ariés,[14] would seem misguided, since even if we will have to die it *does* matter *when* we die: 'I am not sorry to die, since I had to die sometime' (Ariés 1981: 21). Whether defiance will result in a prolongation of life or not is obviously hard to evaluate and we might expect that it has at most marginal value. However, it has been found that defiance, anger or wrath at one's situation might be a source of energy and power in the situation, which of course in many aspects might benefit us.[15]

We saw in relation to cognitive acceptance that Momeyer (1988) argued against denial on the basis of reality contact and, following this, he also supports rebellion against death – or what I would call emotional defiance. Hence, this is done from a more objective view of what makes for a good life and I will take a look at his reasons for rebellion, focusing on the more general objective list reasons for emotional acceptance versus defiance that would support his claims. However, as indicated in the above quotation from Kübler-Ross it does not seem too far-fetched to view denial as, in some cases, a way to defy death, e.g. one way in which teenagers rebel against their parents is simply to ignore their existence.

Following Momeyer it would seem that there are two reasons why we should rebel against or defy death – one has to do with the idea about reality contact, the other with being the right kind of person. Consider the following:

> . . . at the core of the mystique of death acceptance is not resignation to those tragic conditions which render death the lesser evil that may befall one but rather a notion that death may be a positive good . . . the point of the struggle is not to conquer death, but to assert our human-ity, preserve our integrity, and affirm our dignity even in the face of the absurd assault upon them that death presents.
>
> (Momeyer 1988: 10, 13)

Starting with the idea about reality contact, Momeyer argues elsewhere in the book that death is always an evil and at best the least bad of evils in a situation. Assuming that it is good for us to be in contact with reality as it is, how should we respond to such a bad reality? If reality contact is important, to be in contact with reality should probably encompass not only having certain beliefs about this reality but also responding in a proper way to this reality. Then it would seem that we should be in conflict with a bad reality as well as embracing a good reality. That is, to the extent that reality contact makes for a better life we cannot view a bad situation with equanimity: we should defy it. I have argued that death is generally bad for us (even if the least bad of the alternatives at hand) and hence it is something that should be defied on this account of good. On the other hand, I argued above that we should accept a hostility restriction to the idea about reality contact. Does such a restriction fly in the face of Momeyer's argument? I do not think so, because what it implies is that we need not make ourselves aware of a hostile situation, but if we become thus aware we should respond to it with defiance.

Does it make a difference whether defiance results in beneficial results regarding the timing of death? The idea about reality contact being finally good has no such implications. Would it make a difference in relation to Momeyer's second claim about being a certain kind of person? Momeyer explicitly claims that it has not and he uses Camus's *The Plague* to illustrate this. In *The Plague* the protagonist Bernard Rieux continues to fight against the plague in a North African city even if it does not seem to make any difference to the survival of people in the long run (see also Camus's *The Myth of Sisyphtes* where we find a similar theme). Imagine a concentration camp prisoner being brought to the gas chambers, knowing what is about to happen. He also knows, from seeing a large number of other camp prisoners being brought to the gas chambers, that whatever he does there is no chance of escaping his destiny. So defiance will not be instrumentally useful in any way. Would he be worse off if he defied being brought to the slaughter bench (expressing his defiance verbally or by fighting the guards) and better off if he emotionally accepted it? To me it seems, if we accept the idea that it is finally better to be a certain kind of person, that the defiant prisoner is in fact better off (even if the accepting prisoner is understandable). In other words, he is the kind of person we should be in such a case. I think that is what Momeyer's claim amounts to, even if he uses difficult notions such as humanity, integrity and dignity to express it (see the discussion on dignity above). That is, this is the way a proper human being would act or this is worthy of a human being. To preserve integrity would here seem to imply that we act in a way that is in line with the kind of moral and other values we should have.

A bad death outside the concentration camp would not seem to be relevantly different enough (even if different in many other respects) to warrant another attitude. Interestingly, in Israeli hospice philosophy we find support for this defiant attitude to death and acceptance is seen as a case of giving up.[16] It might be argued that there is a relevant difference between the death of a concentration camp prisoner and death from disease, in that the former situation involves death being caused by another human being with the intent of harm, which is not the case in the latter situation. What should be defied is the morally bad act of human killing rather than death itself. Perhaps there is a specific type of badness involved in things inflicted on us by other human beings. Hence, it might be somewhat worse to be murdered than killed by disease. However, the difference in badness would not seem essential to warrant defiance only in the case of badness inflicted on us by other human beings.

Compare a situation in which we are about to die with only a couple of hours left. A longstanding enemy sees his chance to get his revenge and decides to kill us. Is it much worse for us to die by the hand of our enemy than to die a couple of hours later in the disease? It might be somewhat worse since there is someone who resents us enough to kill us in the former case, but it would seem to make only a small difference and our enemy would be deprived of the magnitude of his revenge if he waited that long to kill us. The reason is that what makes killing bad is that we will be dead as a result of it, and what is bad with death (according to the above) is mainly that it deprives us of future good life and a couple of hours does not hurt us that much. So the only real difference (for us, that is, not if we look at other side-effects of the action) would then be that we are resented, which is presumably bad for us. Still, our enemy has resented us for long and just awaited the right moment and hence nothing much is altered as relates to resentment in him killing us. Given this, it would seem strange to claim that we should defy our enemy killing us but not defy death in disease a couple of hours later, even though the badness of the two situations does not differ much.

Hence, accepting the idea about being a certain kind of person, it is likely that we would be better off defying death, apart from any instrumental effects this will have in relation to our lives. Still, we might be reluctant to make such definite claims about human beings in general and how they should be. We could instead relate it to the self-identity of the dying person, something that is at the core of the palliative philosophy according to a number of authors (see, for example, Walter 1994; Field 1996; Seale 1998), and also something that I have argued is essential to a dying person (in the section on dignity). That is, to the extent that I have been the kind of person who has fought and defied what I have found to be bad or if I interpret the defiance as if I am fighting for my life, it might be important for me to continue to do so (Saunders *et al.* 2003). In line with this we might find acceptance, especially if forced upon us by our bodily decay, as a problematic loss of self (Lawton 2000).

It was argued in the above that there might often be a well-being cost to defiance. Does that mean there is a distinct contradiction between the two value approaches? I think what is crucial here is that even if this is the proper attitude to have in front of bad situations, we need not therefore actively seek out such situations and it does not imply that we cannot avoid experiencing such situations to the extent possible. That is, it is not courageous actively to seek out situations of badness just so that we can face them and defy them; instead, that would be foolhardy. Moreover, to the extent that we can reduce the badness of the situation, we have reason to do so as long as it does not imply changing our attitudes or the way we respond to such a situation. Hence, in this character account it is acceptable if we sedate ourselves into avoiding the bad situation, but not if we change the way we respond to the situation. It is partly because we have the proper response in the situation that we need to be sedated. Besides, it is hard to see that remaining conscious at the event of death would be a sign of defiance. It seems we can rage and be in conflict with death and still avoid much of the troublesome well-being effects of facing death in this way.

On the other hand, taking the perspective of people in the vicinity, it might be painful and distressing to watch someone fight and defy the inevitable death (without any results) and it might be better for them if the dying person accepts the fact that she is going to die. A person emotionally accepting death might be easier to handle than a person trying every possible escape route out of her situation and being angry with the fact that she is dying. As Field (1996: 260) expresses it, 'it is difficult to die an overtly angry death in a hospice as the "hospice smile" can be very constraining upon those who want to "rage against the dying of the light"!' In Walter (1994) and in Seale (1998) we also find suggestions that the palliative philosophy would encourage a certain amount of fight or defiance, even if Walter means that this might be restricted to talking about one's anger rather than expressing it. Moreover, Walter voices a possible problem with this view: in explaining people's anger as a normal reaction to impending death rather than seeing it as a reaction to poor care, the personnel might be oblivious to what is really the problem.

However, it might also be painful for people (i.e. the close-ones) to see a person 'give up' in the face of death – especially if he or she has been a fighter before. Hence, from the perspective of people in the vicinity of the dying person it is not obvious what the best attitude is.

Normative aspects of an accepted death

Respect for self-determination should allow patients and close ones to respond to death in any way they like as long as it does not seriously hurt other people. As professional carers we should be able to handle even emotional defiance in a person, even though an emotionally accepting person might be an easier patient. However, the carers must have access to counselling or other professional support to be able to handle the distress that might be caused by dealing with angry and fighting patients. If the dying person or the close one obviously suffers from not accepting death and wants help to come to acceptance, professional carers should of course help to the extent possible.

Again, it is important to be aware of the possible structural aspects and how they affect the patients' ability to express emotional responses of their own choice, i.e. if the care culture favours any of the emotional approaches, especially the more subtle aspects of such an ideology, such as that even if the defying patient is accepted, her death is also generally deemed a worse one.

Self-control in dying

Whether we arrive at the conclusion that we should emotionally accept or defy death, it could be argued that we should be in control of our emotional responses to death.

> It should also be a death marked by consciousness, by a self-awareness that one is dying, that the end has come – but, even more pointedly, a death marked by self-possession, by a sense that one is ending one's days awake, alert, and physically independent, not as a machine-sustained body or a body that has long ago lost its mind and self-awareness . . . I recoil at the prospect of a death marked by pain and suffering, though I hope I will bear it well if that is unavoidable.
>
> (Callahan 1993: 54, 196)

In Callahan self-possession is generally contrasted with control of the external world implied by demands for euthanasia and other measures to control what dying and death will be like (see Smith 2003 for a list of principles for a good death, where control over the external world is the common feature of all principles):[17] 'What has come to count too much is that our choices affect *outcomes* in the world; we are at sea when we cannot do so' (Callahan 1993: 129). What Callahan recommends instead is (partly quoting Viktor Frankl):

> Our human greatness, the sure sign of our transcendence over dumb nature . . . that the self still remains our own, even in its dissolution . . . [the] last of the human freedoms – to choose one's attitude in any given set of circumstances, to choose one's own ways.
>
> (*Ibid.*: 128)

He insists on:

> the strength of the self to choose its stance toward nature rather than feel compelled to dominate it . . . a noble and heroic life can be

achieved by those who have little or no control over the external conditions of their lives, but have the wisdom and dignity necessary to fashion a meaningful life without it.

(*Ibid.*: 99, 126)

In Callahan, to be self-possessed implies not only choosing one's attitude, but choosing a specific attitude, i.e. the more stoical one:[18] 'In another era, we might have embraced fatalism, or a stoicism not far removed from it: accept that which cannot be controlled' (*Ibid.*: 128). It seems that self-possession might be used more or less interchangeably with the less cumbersome expression self-control (which I will henceforth use). In other words, to be self-possessed implies being in control of one's self, or some aspect of our self being in control of some other aspect of us. Following that, we can distinguish between exercising self-control in the weak sense and exercising self-control in the strong sense.

In relation to palliative philosophy, it would seem that the norm would be that we should display or express emotions in the face of death, or at least talk about our feelings even if we should not actually express them to the full (Walter 1994). That is, the above norm about awareness seems to include the norm about talking openly about everything that is related to death and dying, including one's problematic emotions and thoughts. Walter expresses some doubt as to whether we are allowed to express these feelings fully and he voices the view that within the palliative philosophy one might be prone to accept the more 'feminine' display of feelings, e.g. crying, rather than expressions of anger.

When we experience emotional reactions or thoughts that we do not show or make explicit we can be said to exercise self-control in the weak sense: for example, if we feel scared when we enter the scene to give a lecture or if we make a reflection about the audience's lack of intellectual capacity, but do not allow ourselves to show it or let it be shown (which might be difficult taking into account body language). On the other hand, if we could control ourselves to the extent of not feeling scared when entering the scene or not to reflect thus about the audience, we could be said to exercise self-control in the strong sense. The strong version of self-control implies that if we did not exercise such control we *would* feel scared or reflect thus. That is, somewhere under the surface the reaction or thought is lurking and waiting for a weakening of our control.

Hence there is a logical, even if not necessarily an empirical, difference between being self-controlled in the strong sense and being the type of person who does not feel scared when entering scenes (to follow up this example). However, this is a difference that might be very difficult or even impossible to detect (both for the person concerned and for others). For example, if we get scared on a specific occasion, it might be impossible to say whether this is due to temporary loss of control or because that is the kind of situation in which we, being the kind of people we are, do feel scared. The distinction between strong and weak self-control is a matter of degree rather than distinct categories and in the weaker versions we will probably be aware of exercising such control.

What kinds of emotional or cognitive reactions and responses (henceforth emotions and thoughts) do we normally associate with self-control, or would be among the ones that should be controlled according to norms about self-control? We can distinguish between a couple of different aspects. First, it might be because they have a certain character – for example, containing fear or anger – or because they involve a certain evaluation of the situation, such as discontent, envy or superciliousness. Second, they might be too strong – for example, excessive love or excessive fear. In essence, self-control is related to norms for what emotions and thoughts we should show or have in relation to different situations.

In relation to dying, what kind of emotions and thoughts might we experience that could be made the object of self-control? Dying and death would seem to be able to evoke fear, anger, small-mindedness, regret, hate, cowardliness, loss of hope, wishful thinking and a large number of other emotions and thoughts. That is, death and dying seem to be able to evoke a large number and variety of emotions and thoughts. Literature on death and dying supports this claim.[19] Would it make for a better dying to control these responses and reactions – in either the weak or the strong sense?

A possible empirical problem here is that when we are dying, our powers will generally weaken until the point of death and we will probably lose some of our abilities as the dying progresses (Lawton 2000). Consequently, it might be difficult to control the emotions and cognitions we experience, whether in the weak or the strong sense. Callahan (1993: 133) admits to this when he says: 'I do not contend that there can be a total mastery of self and character here, but only that we do have the power to lead ourselves in one general direction or another.' However, let us for now ignore this (highly relevant) difficulty in relation to self-control and assume the dying person to be able to control his or her emotional and cognitional responses and reactions.

Value to the dying person and others

Arguably, a number of different suggestions can be given for why it would make for a better death to be self-controlled: (a) we might avoid the lowering of well-being these emotions and thoughts might cause us, because they might be problematic in themselves but also because they might be instrumentally problematic; (b) in exercising control, we might avoid ruining our close relationships and miss out on the beneficial effects of these; (c) controlling these kinds of responses and reactions in front of death might be the proper way to behave in being the kind of person that it is valuable to be; (d) it might be beneficial to autonomy to exercise control thus. Let us explore these suggestions in turn.

To fear death, be angry at or hate our disease, be disappointed with life, lose hope, find that we loathe the company of our close ones are probably, in most cases, things that will lower our well-being. However, only control in the strong sense would seem to prevent these emotions and thoughts from causing us such a lowering. That is, once we have experienced them they will of course lower our well-being. Not being able to control them strongly, it is often assumed to be better to display them or share them rather than bottle them up (for us, that is). In other words, if we cannot exercise strong control over them it might be better if we do not exercise weak control over them. This would at least be in line with the expressivist idea on emotions, where we should show the emotions that we actually feel in different situations (Walter 1994). However, Walter also notes that in some cases the expression of difficult emotions can cause people to brood on them in a manner that will make them even more problematic.

Someone (of an expressivist bent) might argue that even exercising strong control would be problematic, since these emotions take on another form of expression (i.e. resulting in problematic physical symptoms or even worse psychological symptoms). I will not venture into a discussion of whether this is true or not. Even accepting this, when dying time is scarce and since such reactions are likely to take some time to develop, such a problem does not seem too pressing.

Hence, from a hedonistic perspective we would seem to have reasons to exercise strong control over problematic emotions and thoughts. If this is not possible (and we must remember our weakened status) it is possible to provide reasons both for exercising and for not exercising weak control. Since I am not competent to evaluate whether there is something to expressivism or not, it would seem better to relate it to the individual person and how he or she best handles problematic emotions and thoughts.

In line with this we might also say something about the instrumental problems with not exercising self-control. In much of the Scandinavian culture of which I am a part we are generally cautious about expressing emotions and thoughts. Still, I gather that in any culture people would have difficulties in handling a *full* display of one's inner life. Hence, in any culture there are emotions and thoughts that, if shown, will complicate the relationships in which we are involved and make it more difficult to achieve what we want to achieve (and what is valuable to achieve) in and through these relationships. Primarily, weak self-control would be of essence here. Strong self-control would imply being on the safe side, with less risk of displaying one's inner self by mistake. Walter (1994) has noted the possible conflict here between maintaining social interaction if expressing problematic emotions and thoughts and being held to be insincere (on the expressivist account) if not. But, as he also notes, it might be difficult to distinguish between someone not having any emotions or exercising strong control over them and someone who exercises weak control over them.

It is sometimes argued that we should be able to express whatever we feel and think, but even admitting that (which I am not sure we should), it does not seem empirically possible without complications. So we have a reason to exercise control over what we show to other people if these people are instrumentally important to us and even more so if they have only instrumental value to us. That is, people with whom we do not have a close relationship are likely to be less lenient in relation to emotional and cognitional outbursts. Now, when dying we are likely to be strongly dependent on one group of people, namely carers, and they will be instrumentally important for us to receive good medical management and good care. Once again, it is often argued that professional carers should be able to handle emotional and other outbursts from patients. Still, there is likely to be a discrepancy between the ideal and the reality and a difficult patient (in the above sense) might in fact have some trouble receiving good care. So as patients we might have fairly strong reasons to exercise self-control over our emotions and cognitions in order to receive the best available care. Walter (1994) reports that courage is admired in patients because it seems to make everyone's life easier; and courage would seem to involve some degree of self-control.

However, even if a certain realism about carers leads us to such a conclusion, we have reason to examine critically a practice that cannot handle outbursts of strong emotions and thoughts in the face of death. That is, to claim that patients should be self-controlled in order to fare better in the face of other people might be considered supportive of a morally dubious structure. It might be claimed, and notably some feminists do,[20] that this norm of self-control is a way to exercise power over people for whom emotional and cognitional outbursts are their only way to react against power or oppression or troubling situations. These people simply lack other means of expression or other means to cope with the situation, while the one who is in control or feels in control of what happens to her will have less to gain and more to win in being self-controlled. To be sure, to be self-controlled is to be an easy patient, not to cause trouble to the environment, to adapt to the norms of that environment, and patients like that will generally be easier to take kindly to. Consider the following statement from Glaser and Strauss, a report of sociological studies of care for the dying, in which the personnel's expectations of a 'good' patient are described in a rather ironic tone:[21]

> The patient should maintain relative composure and cheerfulness. At the very least, he should face death with dignity. He should not cut himself off from the world, turning his back upon the living; instead he should continue to be a good family member, and be 'nice' to other

patients. If he can, he should participate in the ward social life. He should cooperate with the staff members who care for him, and if possible he should avoid distressing or embarrassing them. A patient who does most of these things will be respected.

(Glaser and Strauss 1965: 86)

In effect, the norm about self-control, even if instrumentally useful in many cases, might have problematic moral connotations in that it can be used to suppress people who are already in an inferior position.

The second suggestion as to why we should exercise control over emotions and cognitions is that they might damage or ruin intimate personal relationships. Again, it is primarily weak self-control that we are discussing, even if strength might be required in order not to give away emotions and cognitions by mistake. Callahan gives the following suggestion why he found some deaths good or peaceful:

They were the kind of people who had always known when to hold their tongue, to conceal their pain, understanding full well that such a discipline is part of a tolerable life with others . . . If their death were, from the inside, far more terrible than I could know, they hid this well, and thereby made it easier for those of us who survived to face our own deaths better.[22]

(Callahan 1993: 222)

According to an idealized description of intimate personal relationships we should be able to express any emotions or thoughts we have in such a relationship. But, as we all know, this is a highly idealized description and few, if any, relationships can handle such openness without restraints.

To be sure, a close relationship with another human being might result in us getting angry, annoyed, small-minded, envious and supercilious. We might, sometimes, despise the other person, think he is an idiot or just pompous, think we would be better off without this person or something along these lines. It is possible to provide a long list of (problematic) emotions and cognitions that intimate personal relationships might result in. All of them are emotions and cognitions that do not fit very well into the idealized rosy picture of such relationships. I think we can safely say that if we never exercised control over these emotions and cognitions (to the extent that they occur) it would seriously damage and probably ruin the relationship. However, it does not follow from this that we should always exercise control over emotions or thoughts that might crop up in a relationship. For example, if my wife repeatedly does something that annoys me or makes me angry it would seem counter-productive to the relationship to exercise control and not show or give voice to my anger and annoyment. That is, if I am not explicit about how it affects me she will probably continue doing what is problematic (perhaps she will continue anyway, but that is a different story) and it might come to the point where this actually ruins the relationship. There seems to be an abundance of anecdotal evidence of relationships breaking up due to small sources of irritation finally making a hole in the stone. However, control is not an all or nothing affair and we should exercise control to the extent that it will voice what is problematic but not to the extent that it will ruin the relationship (if possible, since a relationship might have reached the point where the only way to change what is problematic is to break it up).

Is this applicable when we are dying? When affected by disease, as most dying persons are, we may be more prone to experience such emotions and cognitions and hence the issue whether to exercise control or not is most definitely an important issue; given that we *can* exercise control following the weakened condition we are in. Now, it might be argued that when someone close is dying we are more prone to accept emotional and other outbursts (and, certainly, should be more prone to do so).

Let us compare this with giving birth. As a husband and father of two children, I know that being present at a delivery might result in being the object of outbursts of anger, fear and a number of other emotions – something that I find rather distressing. Most women are not very self-controlled in the delivery room and as a bystander one will have to stand the display of a number of distressing emotions and cognitions. However to demand that my wife be more self-controlled in such a situation in order to spare me I would find almost outrageous. If I cannot handle or ignore her outburst in a situation that is so distressful to her, it would seem to be my problem rather than hers. Now, dying is likely to be even more distressing than giving birth and hence I would find the same conclusions warranted in dying. Of course, from this it does not follow that such outbursts are excusable or acceptable in just any situation.

Even if one might claim that we should handle such outbursts it is obviously not always the case that we do, and we might even be more sensitive to such outbursts in situations of death and dying. Hence, when dying we might need to consider in what way lack of self-control will actually influence our relationships. On the other hand, if the period of dying is a special time for reconciliation and the resolution of conflicts, it might be instrumentally important to give voice to these conflicts. Conflicts might be voiced in different (more or less hurtful) ways and hence a certain degree of self-control is warranted.

Another reason for exercising self-control is that it is the proper way to behave in the face of (bad) death and dying. However, I have already presented some reasons supporting the suggestion that, given the idea about being in contact with reality or the idea about being a certain kind of person, if death is generally bad it will be proper not to accept such a death emotionally. Whether we have reasons to display this lack of acceptance to other people is a somewhat different question.

Imagine that my daughter or son, God forbid, were killed in a car accident or abused by a child molester or accidentally fell from the top of a cliff. Would it not be improper and a sign of not really grasping the full nature of the situation if I did not show any strong emotions, whatsoever, in relation to such an event? Moreover, would it not have been proper and even a sign of emotional health to show anger, sorrow and remorse. Here it must be noted that the propriety in displaying these emotions does not seem to depend on whether there is a moral agent involved in their death or not, or whether it is the result of the acts of a *malicious* moral agent (even if the exact nature of these emotions might depend on that). Likewise, I do not find any reasons why it would be any less proper when the badness concerns me, rather than someone else.

It is logically possible to acknowledge the true nature of the situation without the above reactions and it is also logically possible to acknowledge the true nature of the situation and exercise strong control over the resulting reactions. However, empirically it would seem difficult to do so when something bad happens to someone we cherish. That is, in order to exercise strong self-control I think we normally have to picture the situation differently from how it actually is.

The only possible alternative where we can be the right kind of person and not experience the above reaction is when we exercise strong control. If we did not react in the above way we would have the wrong kind of personality. So these two items in combination would have it that, since it is difficult to exercise strong control over the reaction that should result from being the right kind of person and acknowledging the true nature of the situation, and since exercising weak control would probably not do us much good if there is anything to hedonism, we could display the above emotions and thoughts when facing situations where we lose something of significant value to us; especially if displaying them will cause them to become less problematic. The loss of our life would seem to qualify as losing something of significant value to us. Once again, we need to be reminded of Walter's comment about the difficulty of judging whether someone is actually feeling something or not in a certain situation. Hence, we should be careful in passing judgement on what someone feels in relation to his or her death on account of what is shown on the outside. However, if there is anything to hedonism we would have reasons to develop or take a drug that would minimise the hedonistic cost of acknowledging the true nature of the situation or being the right kind of person, unless experiencing these emotions has instrumentally important effects on our lives or the lives of other people.

What about the fourth suggestion – that exercising self-control will imply that we are more self-determined? Classically, the idea about self-determination or autonomy implies self-governance in some form, i.e. not being governed by anything outside ourselves or being governed by our true or rational selves. However, first, emotions and cognitions are a part of our selves and hence to be governed by these or not to control these would still seem like self-governance of sorts. Second, even admitting to the fact that we might distinguish between the more and less rational parts or aspects of ourselves, it was implied above that some emotions and cognitions (even the problematic ones) are rational or proper to have in some situations. Still, we might find ourselves overwhelmed by strong emotions and cognitions, seemingly not being able to resist the displaying of them.

Following the account of self-determination given in Chapter 2 we could argue that if displaying or having emotions is not in line with our actual and basic values and desires we are not self-determined in displaying them. So, to the extent that we are overwhelmed by them, we are less self-determined than if we could choose to have and display them whenever we so wanted. From this it does not follow that we are more self-determined every time we exercise self-control in the above sense, since it might be in line with our basic desires to display certain emotions and thoughts. Moreover, our way of relating to emotions and thoughts might be in line with our self-identity, which we have worked on over a number of years, and hence something that is in line with our basic desires about our lives, even if we, as Seale (1998: 129) reports, might be surprised by how we handle oncoming death: 'as a child I know for a fact I was a coward . . . [but now I] find out that in fact, at the last, thank God, you're not actually a coward – I haven't shed a tear since I knew . . . I haven't had a single moment of terror since they told me.' Here it is interesting to note the conflict between the person's self-identity and ego ideal (see the section on consistent death), when he seems to have become what he wanted to become: someone courageous.

Normative aspects of a self-controlled death

Following the discussion there are strong reasons for professional carers to be accepting of people who are not self-controlled in the face of dying and death, unless they are seriously hurtful to other patients and close ones. That is, even if a certain degree of leniency is warranted when patients are abusive to professional carers it is important not to make palliative care into a moral freezone. Not even the dying patient has the right to seriously abuse and hurt other people. On the other hand, they should obviously not influence the dying patient to adopt an expressivist stance when not wanted by the patient.

Facing suffering in dying

In this section I deal with the question of whether there are some sorts of suffering that should be faced rather than delivered from in dying. To be sure, on almost any list of what makes for a good or better death we find the idea that suffering should be kept at a minimum as an essential element. For example, one of the most important goals within all palliative care is the goal of symptom management, where obviously management of pain and suffering is an essential element and it is emphasized that it is not only the physical pain that should be dealt with; instead the talk is of 'total pain' (Saunders and Baines 1983), which includes physical, psychological, social and spiritual[23] aspects. In Weisman's account of an appropriate death it is expressed in the following way: '[The dying person] should be relatively pain-free, his suffering reduced' (Weisman 1972: 39). 'Appropriate deaths are those in which suffering is at a low ebb ... Relief of anguish and resolution of remaining conflicts join in a harmonious exitus' (Weisman 1973: 370).

The central value of well-being would, on the face of it, support the idea that dying without suffering would make for a better dying. But suffering might in some cases be instrumentally beneficial to some good or otherwise necessarily or unavoidably associated with some good. In the literature on good death we often find the idea that some types of suffering are essential or integral to any life.[24] Following such a view, it is argued that this suffering should be dealt with or coped with in a different manner from the sufferings related to physical symptoms. In Callahan the ideas about dying and suffering are voiced in the following manner:

> Pain ordinarily refers to a highly distressful, undesirable sensation or experience ordinarily associated with a physical cause ... Suffering, by contrast, ordinarily refer to a person's psychological or spiritual state, and is characteristically marked by a sense of anguish, dread, foreboding, futility, meaninglessness, or a range of other emotions associated with a loss of meaning or control or both. Not all pain leads to suffering (the pain of the victorious distance runner leads to pleasure), nor does suffering require the presence of physical pain (the anguish of knowing one has Alzheimer's disease) ... Suffering will surely be 'unnecessary' when it serves no purpose, when it is not an inextricable part of achieving important human goals. Unavoidable necessary suffering, by contrast, is that which is the essential means, or accompaniment, of valuable human ends; and not all suffering is.
>
> (Callahan 1993: 95, 97)

Callahan give us some examples of the latter kind of sufferings: 'To take an unpopular position, to stand up for one's rights, to remain true to one's promises and commitments can all entail unavoidable suffering ... the suffering caused by living out one's moral duties or ideals for a life.' (Callahan 1993: 97). Besides the distinction between unnecessary and necessary suffering (or unavoidable suffering, which might not be exactly the same), Callahan distinguishes between the suffering that the medical and caring professions should respond to and the suffering that the suffering person will have to deal with on his or her own, what he calls the two levels of suffering:

> At one level, the principal problem is that of the fear, uncertainty, dread, or anguish of the sick person in coping with the illness and its meaning for the continuation of life and intact personhood ... At a second level, the problem touches on the meaning of suffering for the meaning of life itself. The question here is more fundamental: what does my suffering tell me about the point or purpose or end of human existence, most notably my own?

In practice this will have the following results:

> It means that the doctor should, through counselling, pain relief, and cooperative efforts with family and friends, do everything possible to reduce the sense of dread and anxiety, of disintegration of self, in the face of a threatened death. The doctor should provide care, comfort and compassion. But when the patient says to the doctor that life no longer has meaning, or that the suffering cannot be borne because of its perceived pointlessness, or that a loss of control is experienced as an intolerable insult to a patient's sense of dignity – at that point the doctor must draw a line.
>
> (Callahan 1993: 100–1)

However, Callahan admits: 'What life itself may give us at its end is a death that seems, in the suffering it brings, to make no sense. That is a *terrible* problem, but it is the patient's problem, not the doctor's' (Callahan 1993: 102). These excerpts are taken from a discussion of euthanasia, which Callahan resists on these and other grounds. Without any implications for whether euthanasia should be practised or not or for the role of the physician in relation to the relief of suffering, I will take this as the basis for my discussion of whether there are sufferings in dying that we are *not* better off without.

Before we enter into that discussion it needs to be pointed out that we might have to distinguish between different sufferings on account of the best way to relieve them. That is, some sufferings (most notably physical) are perhaps better relieved by drugs, while others are better relieved by therapy or other measures, which is indicated in the quotations from Callahan (see Brülde 2003 for a discussion on this). There is more to his views than simply that, i.e. he seems to claim that there are sufferings that we should not relieve by any means, even if possible. If we relieve them we will lose something of greater value. In the works of Dame Cicely Saunders we find similar ideas: 'it might be as important to understand the suffering and relate to it and handle it in a creative way as to try to relieve it' (Saunders 1978b: 288). Hence, even if palliative care includes the norm about dealing with the total pain of the dying person, it is not obvious that all suffering or pain should actually be relieved, even if possible.

In this context I will focus on the issue of whether there are cases where a death with some suffering is actually better than a death with no suffering. I will do this by exploring Callahan's ideas, but I will also add a couple of other ideas on when suffering would seem intimately linked to some good and discuss whether they are plausible or not. The important normative aspect of this is whether there are sufferings we should refrain from easing or relieving, and if so, what sufferings and on what grounds.

Value to the dying person and others

Obviously, in any life we are bound to face a certain amount of suffering and hence in that sense suffering is integral to life and will have to be dealt with in any life. However, on the face of it no suffering would seem unavoidable, since it is always possible to be relieved of it by death (i.e. suicide or euthanasia) or by sedation (i.e. terminal or non-terminal). So, to be interesting in this context unavoidable suffering will have to be interpreted to mean that we cannot avoid the suffering without losing something of greater value. This might be expressed as if the suffering is necessarily related or at least strongly related to some good and we cannot have the one without the other. I will take it, and I think both Callahan and Saunders would agree with me, that suffering in itself is bad for us and hence always a cost, even though sometimes a necessary one.

In the following I discuss four suggestions of why suffering might be necessary in relation to some good, see whether it is indeed necessary and evaluate whether the good in question is actually worth the cost (especially given that we are dying). First, it might be a necessary cause or partial cause of something good – as when it is claimed that we need to experience suffering in order to become more genuine, deeper, more profound human beings. Second, it might be a constitutive part of the good in question – as with empathy and compassion, where suffering seems necessary for these emotions to exist. Third, it might be a necessary consequence or risk associated with some good – as when it is claimed that we cannot love someone and not suffer if love goes sour, or Callahan's suggestion that 'To take an unpopular position, to stand up for one's rights, to remain true to one's promises and commitments can all entail unavoidable suffering.' Fourth, it might be unavoidable in the sense of having the same basis as other goods –

for example, both suffering and the enjoyment of close relationships presuppose that we are conscious.

In the first two versions it is supposed we cannot have the good without the suffering, while in the third version we can have the good without actually experience the suffering, since the possible outcome might not be realized. In the fourth version it depends on the extent to which we can get rid of the suffering without affecting the common basis, which is normally consciousness. Are there any cases where we cannot have a good without experiencing the suffering and, moreover, would we actually get a worse death if we relieved the suffering – even if it takes more draconian measures like euthanasia or sedation (Tännsjö 2003)?

Consider the following quotation from William Arrowsmith, found in Callahan (1993: 125): 'with the loss of suffering comes also the loss of dignity and *sophia* [wisdom]. For it is in the struggle with necessity that heroism is born'. Obviously, some people do become more profound and heroic as a result of suffering.[25] However, people do also become bitter and mean as a result of suffering. Hence, suffering is not always ennobling.[26] In Lawton's vivid descriptions of dying patients in a hospice it is hard to find anything ennobling in the suffering they experience; it is something that leads to a loss of their selves rather than to profundity (Lawton 2000). Besides, is it really the experience of suffering that makes us more profound, or is it going through the situations that result in suffering?

Consider the following situation. A man loses his daughter in a tragic accident and experiences suffering as a result of this. This event makes him rethink his life, realizing that instead of spending time with his children he has spent his time working, reading crime stories and renovating his house. As a result he starts to make other priorities, realizing what is of more lasting value. In a sense, he becomes more profound. However, it was not the suffering *per se* that made him rethink his life but losing his daughter, and had it been possible to escape the suffering (by some drug or whatever) he would probably still have reconsidered his life. In other words, it is not handling the suffering, i.e the experiences of 'anguish, dread, foreboding, futility, meaninglessness', that makes us more profound but handling the situation that results in our suffering, though the suffering might make us somewhat more motivated to reconsider our lives in order to get rid of the suffering. However, if we reconsider our lives to get rid of the suffering we will stop, not necessarily when we have become more profound, but at the point where our suffering is eased. Moreover, often we start to reconsider our lives after the worst suffering has passed.

It is reasonable to assume that we might become deepened and more profound without experiencing any suffering or even troubling situations – for example, by character training, a life devoted to serious thinking or more positive experiences (for example, having children). Following this, I am far from convinced that suffering is indeed necessary in order to become a deeper and more profound human being, even if it might be the case that we can become more profound as a result of experiencing certain situations of which suffering is often also a result.

Even if we do accept this idea, is it so obvious that profundity is worth a lot of suffering, since suffering would seem an obvious evil on any account of good, while profundity has more doubtful value? I, for one, would rather keep my daughter and remain shallow. This would be even more pertinent at the end of life when we would seem to have even less reason to become more profound. Moreover, as argued in Badham (1996: 112), if we really accept this idea we should probably be more restrictive with all form of analgesics, something I think most of us have a hard time accepting. Hence, if we cannot escape suffering or the situations that lead to suffering we have reasons to try to make something good of it (to the extent possible), but that does not imply that this good is actually worth the suffering.

Another idea is that it is necessary to experience suffering in order to appreciate life to the full. This would lead to the somewhat absurd situation that if we really value our lives, we should not do anything to reduce the suffering that life results in, since that would indicate that we do not value life enough. Drawing this to the extreme, someone putting up with a whole life of suffering would seem to value life immensely in comparison to someone trying to reduce any suffering her life results in.

Possibly, if someone continues to live a life full of suffering when suffering cannot be reduced, he might do this as a result of valuing his life. However, he might also do it because he fears death, adapts to the strict norms concerning suicide in society or thinks he deserves it, or whatever. That is, there might be reasons for putting up with a life full of suffering besides valuing life. Moreover, if we put up with suffering even when it is possible to be relieved from it, this would be an indication of disvaluing our lives. It is more plausible that the reason is that we think we deserve suffering, want to punish ourselves or think we are not worthy of having our suffering relieved. I would fail to understand someone claiming to endure suffering because he highly values his life in such a case. Furthermore, if there is something to hedonism suffering reduces the value of a life, and hence from such a perspective we would end up in the paradoxical situation that he is willing to reduce the value of his life in order to affirm the value of it. Once again, it does not seem impossible to appreciate life without experiencing suffering (it would even seem more proper to appreciate life without having to experience suffering to arrive at such an appreciation). A similar line of reasoning could, I propose, be made in relation to any other suggestion for good things, where suffering is supposed to be a necessary cause (partial or not).

In the second case the latter option would not be open, even in a hypothetical case, since suffering is supposed to be a constitutive part of the good. In relation to dying and death it could be argued that unless we suffer we would not give other people the opportunity to be empathetic or compassionate towards us, and unless other people suffer we would not have the opportunity to be empathetic and compassionate towards them. Hence, in removing suffering we would 'jeopardize . . . the kind of community that furthers its members' capacity to bear one another's suffering . . . and enter a claim to change the nature of human relationships' (Callahan 1993: 116). Even if empathy and compassion undoubtedly are good attitudes to adopt to someone suffering and a good way to be as a person, that does not seem to make up for the suffering and, on the whole, we would be better off without the suffering (even if we thereby also lost the empathy and compassion). Further, I am not sure that we should accept suffering just to allow *other* people to benefit from being empathetic or compassionate towards us. That is, such a sacrifice on behalf of the dying person might be chosen, but from the perspective adopted here it does not necessarily add to the goodness of the dying person's life. I am even less sure that we should *demand* such a sacrifice on behalf of dying people just to enable other people to be empathetic and compassionate.

According to the third case, suffering is a necessary consequence or risk of some good. However, depending on whether the suffering is synchronic with the good or not it might still be avoidable. That is, if suffering is an outcome of a good in the sense of following (timewise) the good and hence is diachronic with the good, it seems possible to avoid it. However, if the suffering is coexistent with the good and we cannot get rid of the suffering without at the same time getting rid of the good, suffering is obviously unavoidable.

Is this actually the case with dying and death? Given the state of the world, life will necessarily result in death, but death is diachronic in relation to life and in death we do not experience any suffering – hence life versus death does not seem to be a case of this. However, as dying has been defined in this context, a period of dying necessarily precedes any event of death and to the extent that we are aware that we are dying or if dying is associated with problematic physical symptoms we will most often experience suffering. Still, suffering is not a necessary outcome of the good of life: first, some people die instantly without having experienced a prior period of suffering; second, we might also deny the fact that we are dying and so avoid suffering, at least the suffering that is more directly associated with losing one's life.

Moreover, if there is a necessary suffering as an outcome of life a good candidate would be the suffering caused by physical decay and disease in dying. However, I have not found anyone arguing that we should not try every possible means to relieve that kind of suffering. So why should we treat the suffering resulting from losing one's life differently? Besides, any such suffering (to the extent synchronic with the good in question) will have to be weighed against such a good to see whether the suffering is outweighed by this good. It seems that is an open question that will have to be answered in each particular case.

In consequence, it seems that suffering is an almost necessary result of dying to the extent that we value our lives. However, it is hard to see how such suffering actually makes our dying better and we seem to have as strong a reason to relieve such suffering as that resulting from physical decay (which would seem an even more necessary consequence of dying).

This is what seems to be implied in the following quotation from Callahan (1993: 100–1): 'when the patient says to the doctor that life no longer has meaning, or that the suffering cannot be borne because of its perceived pointlessness, or that a loss of control is experienced as an intolerable insult to a patient's sense of dignity'. Hence, if life is not worth living at this point it would be better ended. If so, suffering is not an unavoidable consequence of some good (since there is no good left that will be lost if we end the suffering) and we could end the suffering without losing a life worth living. On the other hand, if life is worth living despite the suffering then suffering is still not intimately linked to a good life because if we could relieve this suffering in other ways than by ending the person's life we would make the person's life better. This moves us on to the fourth suggestion, which I think is the one most pertinent to our discussion.

Suffering might be related to other goods in sharing the same basis and we cannot get rid of the one without the other. Obviously the best suggestion for this basis is consciousness. Hence, when the only way to relieve suffering is through reduction of consciousness we jeopardize every good that is dependent on us being more or less fully conscious and we will have to balance the cost of suffering against the cost in terms of losing other goods. In the words of Callahan (1993: 52), 'The same consciousness that allowed for a tame death, alert to the end, could also, under less favorable circumstances, make possible an awareness of the pain of a last, fatal, illness.' Still, it is not a given fact that it is always better to remain conscious and suffer than to get rid of the suffering and lose some other goods at the same time. This will depend on the balance between the good and the suffering in question.

Summary

In summary, I side with Callahan to the extent that he argues for a death without suffering generally being a better death. On the other hand, I find it more doubtful whether there are sufferings that are intimately linked to a good apart from having the same basis, i.e. consciousness. That is, it is questionable whether there are cases where we would lose something if we were able to reduce or relieve our suffering as far as it does not also involve a reduction in consciousness. Hence, I have found no reason to believe that there are sufferings that we in principle should not try to relieve in dying. Still, it would be foolish not to distinguish between different sufferings when it comes to effective methods of treatment or relief.

Normative aspects of a death without suffering

Given the above discussion it seems reasonable to respect the self-determination of the patient as far as possible and go along with the patient's views on the value of suffering in dying. To the extent that a patient decides that the suffering is great enough to outweigh the value of being conscious at the end of life, she should be offered terminal sedation.

It is important to note that the patient might have a moral obligation to close ones, which of course might turn either way. That is, it might give her reason to endure a certain suffering (at least for some time). But it might also give her reason to relieve the suffering if the close ones find it difficult to see her suffer. Here it is important to emphasize that the close ones should then be in a situation where the actions of the patient would have severe effects on their good life, effects that might not be dealt with in other ways, since we should be extremely wary of overriding a patient's views on her own suffering. In the case of a patient who does not want to have her suffering relieved, an alternative for her close ones is to avoid the patient.[27]

Conclusions and relevance to palliative care

In this chapter we have discussed whether we have reason to face death in a particular manner. More specifically, do we have reason to face death acquainted with death, aware of death, accepting death, self-possessed or suffering.

In relation to acquaintance with death it was argued that my prior acquaintance with death does little to make dying easier for me when I am dying myself. This might not be very relevant to palliative care, since when we face palliative care it is probably too late to get acquainted with death in a way that would be workable anyway. Still, the scarce support for prior acquaintance should be reason enough not to expose me unnecessarily to the death (or problematic dying) of other people even when in palliative care. However, we found support for the idea that my prior acquaintance with death might enable me to handle better the death of other people, especially in situations when I am not personally involved. In effect, this would constitute support for palliative care as such, where carers are well experienced in facing the death and dying of people.

In relation to awareness of death a number of reasons why we should be aware of oncoming death were explored and none of these was found to have unambiguous support. The strongest argument was that awareness is necessary to take steps to avoid otherwise premature death, which was questioned, since that does not necessarily involve awareness that we are dying.

That awareness is necessary to make certain preparations. However, the strength of this argument was found to depend on whether these preparations are important enough to warrant the problematic awareness of oncoming death and also whether they do presuppose awareness of death in the vicinity of death. That awareness of death might make the time left more valuable was found to have some support, but once again the strength of this argument depended on whether the priorities we make as a result of this would not be made anyway and whether they actually bring that much more value to our lives. That awareness would be beneficial to our relationships was found to have ambiguous support, even if it seems reasonable that a joint attitude, whether awareness or denial, would be the best.

Hence, whether awareness is beneficial to a good death was found to depend on what we find important in life and what we need to control: whether it is important that we are able to continue to live the kind of life we have lived and maintain hope, or to fashion the last days in a specific manner. If we want to find a stronger reason for awareness than what fits best with our own way to live, it was argued that we might have moral reasons to become aware of oncoming death when not doing so will cause our close ones serious trouble.

It seems that the discussion about awareness of death is highly relevant to palliative care, as is shown by the number of articles discussing this aspect of a good death by far outweighing the discussion of any other of the ideas discussed in this context. It seems obvious that the idea about awareness of death making for a better death still has a strong hold within palliative care, both in literature and in my own experience when facing palliative carers. Hence, we need to discuss the issue of awareness further within palliative care, in order that it will not become an inherent norm for how all palliative patients should relate to their oncoming death.

In relation to acceptance of death it was argued, as in relation to awareness, that acceptance of death gets ambiguous support to a large extent depending on what theory of value we accept. From a more hedonistic standpoint we might be better off accepting death but from the perspective of being a certain kind of person or from reality contact we might, on the other hand, be better off defying death. This is again relevant to palliative care, since acceptance is, to some extent, on a par with awareness when it comes to norms for how to face death within palliative care, and we need to have a critical discussion of whether it is the best attitude to adopt for all dying people.

In relation to self-possession it was argued that, following the above, it gets ambiguous support and we did not find any conclusive reasons for why we should be self-possessed rather then not when at the end of life. The strongest reason is a moral one, i.e. to spare other people from getting seriously hurt by what we do. However, it was also claimed that we should have a fairly large tolerance of dying people's ways of facing death. This discussion is also relevant to palliative care, both since people within such care will face death differently with regard to self-control or self-possession and since we saw that we might find more definite norms about how people should face or behave in the face of death and we need to discuss whether these norms actually voice the best way, generally, to face death.

In relation to suffering it was claimed that all suffering is in itself bad, and something we have strong reasons to minimize unless it has good instrumental consequences. However, it was argued that none of the suggestions for why suffering would have such instrumental value could be strongly supported. As a general rule we will always have strong reasons to ease the suffering of the dying patient, whatever causes his suffering, and it is only the dying patient who could judge whether easing his suffering could risk something else of value. The best bet for when this could be the case is when easing the suffering will imply affecting the consciousness of the patient to the degree that other things, depending on being conscious, will be affected. This is highly relevant to palliative care, since symptom management and relief of suffering is at the heart of the palliative philosophy.

In effect, the discussion can be said to result in the general conclusion that we do not find strong support for any specific way to face death and we might have reason, depending on circumstances and our own values, to face death in a number of different ways.

Notes

1 See, for example, Gorer (1955), Kübler-Ross (1969, 1974), Feigenberg (1979), Elias (1985), Walter (1993), Edgar (1996b), Longaker (1996) and Smith (2000).
2 See, for example, Elias (1985), Walter (1994), Ballard (1996) and Seale (1998).
3 See, for example, McNamara *et al.* (1994).
4 I owe this point to Professor David Clark.
5 I owe this point to Niklas Juth.
6 See Glaser and Strauss (1965: 40–1) for a discussion of how patients manage to do this (see also Field 1996).
7 See Glaser and Strauss (1965: 43), Field (1996) and Lawton (2000).
8 Retold by Professor Astrid Norberg in a lecture.
9 See also Saunders (1978a), Ariés (1981), Saunders and Baines (1983), Callahan (1993), McNamara *et al.* (1994) and Janssens (2001). In a European survey made in relation to the European project PALLIUM (palliative care ethics), 92.7 per cent of the palliative care personnel deemed acceptance of human mortality an important concept within palliative care (Janssens 2001).
10 See, for example, Lundin (in Beck-Friis and Strang 1995).
11 See Ariés (1981) and Badham (1996: 107).
12 See Kübler-Ross (1969), Larsson (1984), Grennert and Grützmeier (both in Beck-Friis and Strang 1995). In Momeyer (1988) this is referred to as 'death mystique'.

13 See Ballard (1996: 21ff) on this, where he also quotes the emotional acceptance of Marcus Aurelius: 'Do not despise death, but be well content with it, since this too is one of the things which nature wills.'

14 See also Fredriksson-Örndahl (1987) and Twycross (1995).

15 Clary Berg in a personal message about her forthcoming thesis reporting on research in relation to women with breast cancer.

16 See Edvardson (1984) and Samson Katz (1993).

17 See also Glaser and Strauss (1965: Chapter 5).

18 See, for example, Nussbaum (1994: Chapters 9–12) for a discussion of the stoic attitudes.

19 See, for example, Doyle et al. (1998), Ellingson and Fuller (1998) and Lawton (2000).

20 See, for example, Lehtinen (1998: Chapter 7).

21 My own experiences from more recent care do not wholly contradict this picture.

22 Following the discussion on acquaintance with death we might be somewhat sceptical about the latter claim here and being 'deceived' thus might make our own dying come as an unpleasant surprise.

23 In the Swedish context the concept 'spiritual' is often replaced by the less religious concept 'existential' (see, for example, SOU 2001).

24 See Saunders (1978b), Saunders and Baines (1983), Ahlbäck et al. (1998), Öhlén (2000) and Janssens (2001).

25 Longaker (1996) argues that we should, indeed, use suffering to our advantage in this way when we have to face it, i.e. make a virtue out of necessity.

26 See Badham (1996) for a similar criticism of the Christian version of this idea.

27 However, in de Marinis (1998) we find an example of a Muslim woman who refused pain management in the belief that it would solve the relational conflicts within her family and, as a matter of fact, they were solved.

Prepared to die

This chapter deals with some of the preparations we are supposed to make before we die in order to get a good death and whether these preparations should be made in a specific way. The preparations dealt with in this context are the kind of preparations we are supposed to have stronger reasons to make when about to die than otherwise in life. We will start by looking at the idea that we should prepare for death in a specific manner, i.e. according to some ritual. Then we will take a look at the ideas about closure, about making an end-review of life and about staging one's departure.

Rituals in dying

It has been argued that in order to get a better or easier or simpler death we would benefit from having rituals to follow in dying. For example, in the writings of the French sociologist and historian Philippe Ariés it is argued that we have lost something of value when there are no well established rituals in relation to dying and death. In his account the simplicity of death refers primarily to the existence of ritualized practices surrounding death: 'The acts performed by the dying man, once he has been warned that his end is near, have a ceremonial, ritual quality' (Ariés 1981: 18). It also refers to the fact that death had certain unchanging features before the rise of modern medicine. However, even if the process of dying and event of death have been made longer and more complex and variable by the progress of medicine (though this is questioned by some: see Seale 2000), we are unlikely to want to buy constancy at the cost of shorter lives and more painful dying processes. Hence, I will focus on the other simplifying aspect in Ariés's writings, i.e. the ritual quality of what is done by the dying man (or woman).

At this point it is important to distinguish between having a ritual for doing something, having a formula for doing something and just doing something. Let me exemplify this with the action of getting dressed. When I put on my clothes I might just do it without any particular idea of how and in what order to do it, apart from the order related to function. That is, I start with the underwear in no particular order and then put on the rest of my clothes in no particular order, and the order in which I put on my clothes might change from day to day. Sometimes I start with my socks and sometimes I end with my socks. However, I might also do it according to a formula, mine or someone else's, i.e. I always start with the socks, and then move on to my underwear, trousers and shirt in that order, and there might be good reasons to chose one formula before another. Still, it is not a ritual but only a formula for how to dress. To make it into a ritual something more is needed, i.e. that following the formula is imbued with a symbolic meaning apart from what is inherent in what I actually do (Seale 1998). For example, if I were a priest my dressing into my priestly gown would be a ritual, since the different clothes are supposed to symbolize different aspects of the Christian faith. In this section I focus on the ritual aspects of what we might perform in dying, not on what is done or said *per se*. That is, I focus on a ritualized way to prepare to die, not on the preparations as such, which to some extent will be dealt with later.

Rituals are obviously often closely associated with religious practices, including when they concern death and dying (Walter 2003), and it is easy to use religious examples when illustrating rituals. However, much of what we do in normal life could be characterized as ritual, since it is imbued with symbolic meaning. An example is when we take someone's hand with the symbolic meaning of welcoming or greeting her or when we hoist a piece of cloth (better known as a flag) in order to symbolize celebration or nationalism (Goffman 1967). The meaning aspect of rituals will imply that they are basically social entities, since meaning is an essentially social entity (Walter 1994). That is, rituals will normally be socially instituted, regulated and enforced and even if I could ascribe a certain symbolic meaning to what I do and hence make up a new ritual, it will take some time before the actions are imbued with such a meaning for me and even longer before they will become a ritual with such a symbolic meaning for other people. However, before my self-invented action or series of actions becomes a ritual it will be a formula for what to do.

It has been argued that hospice culture as such could be interpreted as a rite or ritualized way to handle the passage from the living over the dying to the dead, drawing on the discussion about 'rites of passage' (Froggatt 1997; see also Field 1996, observing the lack of such rituals or rites in relation to death and dying). However, in this context I will not discuss this interesting meta-interpretation of hospice culture as such, but focus on more limited rituals that could be relevant to death and dying; that is, the kind of rituals that might regulate specific preparations relevant to death and dying, not the dying process as such.

Rituals might not only be *just a* way or *the best* way to do or express certain things, but might even be essential to achieve a certain outcome or result (or at least thought to be essential). The legal ritual to follow in order to get married can be said to be an example of a ritual where the marriage will not take place if the ritual is not adhered to. To take another example, if the ritual of communion is not followed (for example, if the bread and wine are not consecrated) we have not received communion by eating a piece of bread and drinking some wine. Hence, in some cases the ritual is essential in arriving at the result the ritual is supposed to be furthering. However, if we disregard the case of religious rituals, where we might believe that the ritual is instituted by God and cannot be changed without losing out as a result, or where we in changing the ritual would not be doing the thing in question any more, it seems far-fetched to believe that there are secular cases where following the ritual is actually the only possible way to do or express the thing in question. Even if following the legal formula for marriage is essential in relation to a certain legal system, it is not difficult to imagine another system where we follow another formula or ritual and still get married – just compare such formulas in other cultures. Hence, in this context I will boldly assume that the rituals we are discussing are not of an essential character, i.e. they are not the only possible way to achieve the good presumably associated with them, even though they might be the best way.

Value to the dying person and others

Following this, why is it better (for us) to do and express things in a ritualized manner or why is it better (for us) if a certain practice is ritualized? The label provided by Ariés gives us a hint as to why it would be better, i.e. it is supposed to make this practice or the doing or expressing of these things simpler in some ways. In other words, in having a ritual we will know what to do. However, this would seem true even of what I have called having a formula for what to do, i.e. having a chart of what path to follow even if such a formula does not have any symbolic meaning. So, let us take a look at what a ritual might contribute and compare it with having formulas for what to do to see whether it might be helpful enough to have such a formula, even if it is not a ritual.

Apart from giving us a chart for what to do in a specific situation the ritual provides us with a means to express something with what we do. So if we adhere to the ritual of etiquette at dinner parties we will not only know what to do, e.g. what fork to use, how to eat the soup, how to respond to the other guests (for example, how to make a toast or carry on a conversation), how and when to express appreciation, how to dress; we will also express something with the rituals we follow, first something about ourselves, e.g. that we are well bred, that we are the kind of persons well fitted into the more privileged classes or whatever. But we will also express something with the rituals; for example, by making a toast we express appreciation or salute someone, by avoiding embarrassing conversations we express delicacy and respect for our dinner company. All of this might obviously be beneficial to our and other people's well-being, since we will not feel awkward or lost in the situation and we will not upset other people or make them feel awkward. It might also enable us to succeed with projects and plans that are dependent upon the people we associate with. Moreover, we will have means to express or signal what kind of background we have or what kind of person we are, or express respect and appreciation.

However, this presupposes that we are well acquainted with and have internalized these rituals, so that they come naturally to us. If we have not, we will not as easily benefit in the above manner. To the extent that these rituals are important in the situation, we might find it negative not being able to live up to them, perhaps even being the object of other people's sanctions, and the rituals will not make things easier for us. At least, we will clearly show that we do not belong to the same category of people as the other dinner guests, something that might have negative consequences for us. This is a problem to the extent that we worry about what other people think about us, or worry about being liked by other people, something most of us do, and also to the extent that we are dependent upon these people to succeed with our plans and projects. Moreover, our perhaps more spontaneous ways of showing appreciation and respect might make people feel embarrassed or be misinterpreted. On the other hand, we might also consciously break the norms to express disrespect or mark our distance from the rest of the group, which presupposes that we are familiar with these norms to some extent.

Would a formula do the trick in this situation? A formula would give a clue as to what to do, without being expressive of something beyond it being such a clue. However, would we really have any reason to have such a clue? If no one bothered about what fork we used or in what way we ate our soup or that we should avoid certain conversations, could we not just take it by ear? That is, a formula might be needed when we find ourselves afraid or negatively insecure in the face of what we should do in the situation, but also when there are better or worse ways to handle the situation. In other words, we might have good reasons always to use a spoon when eating soup, even if we are not sanctioned for using the fork and using the spoon does not really express anything apart from it being a good means to finish our soup before it gets cold. A ritual might have evolved based on considerations of the best way to handle a certain situation given certain values, but is generally given a more fundamental status than as just the best way to handle this situation, and is hence also often associated with sanctions. This more fundamental status is likely to be closely associated with the symbolic meaning that the ritual expresses, and the value ascribed to what it expresses. Hence, in relation to a ritual we might be sanctioned not only for not handling the situation in the best way but also for not expressing its meaning or expressing it in an improper way. In relation to a formula we might only be sanctioned for the first of these, which of course might be negative enough. Still, formulas that are well established would often seem to become rituals, since they will start to express something beyond themselves and we will provide them with a background narrative to support them, something that might easily make them into rituals.

Rituals (and formulas) are problematic not just because they require that we are well acquainted with them; they might also regulate behaviour in a less than ideal way. To return to our dinner party, the rituals of etiquette prescribe that we should avoid embarrassing issues in conversations, we should not discuss politics unless we know the other person to sympathize with us, we should not discuss the problem of world starvation when the main course is being served. It might be questioned whether this is actually the best way to behave at dinner parties. From a well-being perspective it might be, but from the perspective of being a certain kind of person or from the perspective of reality contact we should probably not avoid important issues just because they cause inconvenience or embarrassment. Perhaps we even have a moral reason to cause embarrassment or make people feel awkward under certain circumstances; for example, when in the company of bigots. Another problem with rituals and formulas is that they are detrimental to spontaneity and freedom and might also hide the important essence of what we are doing. In the religious context, a reaction to ritualized prayer might be that it does not give us the opportunity to express spontaneously what we actually think and feel in relation to God. Moreover, we might follow the ritual more by habit than by heart and hence avoid a more sincere or authentic response.

To summarize, rituals have the benefit of providing us with a preformulated way to handle the situation and also a way to express a certain meaning through our way of handling the situation, something that might give us a sense of security and confidence. Rituals might also give us a way to achieve other things we value, to the extent that such an expression is instrumental to this. On the other hand, rituals require that we are well acquainted with them and might also be associated with sanctions for not following them. Moreover, they might not be the best way to achieve important values in the situation and they might also hinder spontaneity and sincerity. Formulas will provide us with most of the benefits of rituals, except for being expressive of a further meaning. On the other hand, it is likely that formulas are less well established (since formulas tend to become rituals after a while) and hence less associated with sanctions and more open for revision. At the same time, they suffer from similar problems as rituals in possibly hindering spontaneity and sincerity. Obviously unregulated or less regulated behaviour might leave us lost as to what to do but gives us the opportunity to act more spontaneously and perhaps also with greater sincerity (perhaps it is important to show that we actually are lost in the situation). Are these conclusions relevant in relation to rituals in dying and death?

It was claimed that the advantages of having and following established rituals seem to be things like feeling at ease in the situation, not having to spend effort pondering how to behave in that situation, making other people feel comfortable in the situation and having a way to make sense of and express adherence to some greater context in the situation. This is obviously applicable in relation to dying and death, as Daniel Callahan (1993: 33) expresses it: 'the comfort of knowing how to behave publicly in the presence of death'. Let us assume that when we are dying we should do the following things (all found in Ariés in different forms): we should gather people important to us, we should sort out all of our affairs with these people, we should distribute our belongings among them, we should say a proper goodbye to each and every one of them.

Obviously, to make all these things takes time and effort and, given the possibly shorter trajectories of dying and death in earlier times,[1] having a ritual would have helped us perform them all. The lack of time would also have left us little time when not knowing what to do. In effect, it might have brought us confidence in knowing what to do and lacking the time to think too much about what death implied. On top of this it seems plausible that people in the vicinity would also have felt secure knowing that the dying person followed these rituals and would not upset them or make them feel awkward. Nor would they have been negatively surprised, since what would happen was mapped out in advance. So, given the trajectory of earlier deaths, there were probably some well-being benefits in having and observing rituals on top of the value in doing the preparations in question. However, similar reasons could be given for having a formula for what to do, even if it was argued above that it is likely that a formula would not have been as well established and socially agreed upon as a ritual is likely to be, and the adherence to a formula would not express belonging to a certain context in the same way as a ritual is likely to do. Hence the benefits for bystanders might not be as pertinent with a formula as with a ritual.

A problem in relation to the more extended nature of dying is that we do not have to follow rituals or formulas in order to use time optimally and even a large set of rituals or formulas will not be capable of keeping the dying person busy up to her death, and hence there will still be time left for thinking about death, for being lost or at odds about what to do. Perhaps this is to overstate the problem since we might imagine that in having a set of rituals or formulas to follow at the end of life we might confidently await the time when these should be implemented. The value of the ritual or the formula is to provide us with a plan or path to follow on our way to death.

However, if we are not well acquainted with these rituals or formulas and they do not come naturally to us, we are not likely to benefit in this way. It might be troubling trying to follow them and we might experience embarrassment and even shame when failing to do so. Besides, it would not seem to be of essential importance how we behave publicly in the presence of death. If people do not expect us to behave in a specific way we might not be worse off for not knowing how to behave (if there is a proper way to behave, something that might be questioned). On the face of it, the good could as well or better be achieved in other ways than by following a set of rituals or formulas; for example, by spending time with close ones, by having counselling or by indulging in some attention- and time-consuming interest (Walter 1994). What is essential here is the extent to which we are benefited from knowing beforehand what to do and to what extent it is important to us to express belonging to a greater context or not.

As indicated above, it might also be the case that the rituals, with their symbolic expressions, hide the true essence of the situation of dying and death. In the words of Callahan (1993: 33): 'There can be nothing worse than concocted, self-conscious ritual, creating a make-believe world of sweetness and light to cover the harshness of death.' Furthermore, people will be restricted as to what options they will have and it might hinder spontaneity and a more genuine response to the situation. For example, it might be better to think about death without using any preset formulas for this, as might be the case if we spend time observing rituals. Given that death is indeed bad for us, perhaps we should not take comfort in dying or comfort others in dying but (with Dylan Thomas 1952) 'rage against the dying of the light'.

A considerable problem with rituals in relation to dying and death is that there are no rituals of the well established kind in society today. That is, the idea about a common and shared meaning of death would seem to be an idea lost in our pluralistic society (Walter 1994; Seale 1998). In Elias (1985) it is claimed that the old traditions and rituals probably seem shallow and worn-out to people today and an emphasis on informality and spontaneity in our (Western) society makes it hard to establish new rituals. To elaborate on this, what made rituals work in the old days (if indeed they did) was probably that they were adopted not only by the person dying but by all surrounding him, that there was a social pressure to follow them and that the idea of alternatives was not at hand.

Consequently, it is doubtful whether we would actually benefit from establishing a new set of rituals, especially since it would be difficult to establish new rituals and make them become rituals with which we are well acquainted. In effect, the idea about establishing individualized or group-orientated rituals that we find in Clark and Seymour (1999) would not seem to be an idea that it is possible to realize (see also Walter 1994). What we could do is to come up with individualized or group-oriented formulas for what to do, i.e. a plan of what to do and in what order to do it at the end of life, formulas that might evolve into rituals if they get a hold on people and are socially transferred and upheld. However, this will obviously take some time and the dying person coming up with the formula cannot benefit from it as a ritual. Still, a formula might be good enough and give us the benefits we are after in striving for new rituals.

Perhaps a reason why some people want to ritualize death is that rituals are normally associated with more solemn occasions and we want to give dying and death such an aura. If so, a version of Callahan's comment above might be relevant, i.e. that we should not create a make-believe world of solemnity, hiding the badness of death. Moreover, some rituals might even be positively detrimental to the dying patient. Loewy and Springer Loewy (2000: 56) argue that technology might be used as modern rituals:

> People often look upon these efforts today in much the same way as last rites used to be (and for some people still are) looked upon – as symbolic efforts. They are symbols that we often feel are everyone's dues, symbols that represent a proper death and symbols that comfort those left behind.

In such a case, if technology unduly prolongs the life of the patient or distorts his dying in a negative sense, it will be problematic and we should probably find less problematic ways to seek comfort as close ones. (See Chapter 6 for a further discussion of the use of technology.)

Normative aspects of a ritualistic death

Because of the ambiguous support for rituals it seems that we have to leave it up to the dying patient and close ones to decide whether there are any rituals they should follow – and, if so, support them. Moreover, we should be careful, given the above discussion, to internalize a ritualized behaviour in relation to death and dying within the palliative care philosophy. That is, such an internalized ritual might function as a structural straitjacket on patients within palliative care.

On the other hand, to help dying persons and their close ones to try to map out their path to death in advance might be helpful for some. Hence, care personnel have strong reasons to help patients and their close ones with this and also to help them to follow the map to the extent that it still fits the terrain.

Completion of worldly affairs

A more substantial type of preparation supposed to bring along a better death is that we complete or conclude our worldly affairs.[2] Before evaluating this idea we need to spell out more clearly what might be meant by worldly affairs and, moreover, what it implies to complete or conclude them or to bring them to a closure.

In using the term 'worldly affairs' I want to distinguish this alleged feature of good death from the things that characterized the *Ars Moriendi* tradition, where the focus was more on completing religious affairs. The term refers to the economic projects or transactions that we are involved in, our professional projects, our personal projects and our societal projects. To give a sense of what these different projects might imply it is sufficient to give a few examples. Our financial investments, the property we own, the loans we have taken or the things we have signed up to buy are examples of the economic projects and transactions we are involved in. The philosophical treatise on a good dying we are writing, the house we are building or the management job we have might be examples of professional projects (but they might also be personal projects or both). The sport we are trying to excel in or the character we are developing might be examples of personal projects. Finally, the Church we are members of, the political party we are working for or the protest movement we are fighting for might be examples of societal projects (as well as personal and perhaps also professional projects). These are examples of the rather wide range of worldly affairs that we might refer to when claiming that our worldly affairs should be completed or concluded or brought to a closure before we die.

It is not difficult to imagine someone having a large number of such projects going on at the time she enters the period of dying (perhaps even more so when in the 'prime' of life). Hence, due to lack of time (and energy) we would want to know if it is indeed good to complete these affairs and, if so, whether some are more important to complete than others.

However, before moving on to the value discussion, we need to say something about what it would mean to complete these affairs, if indeed they can be completed. Completion has to do with the way we finish things and might be distinguished from other ways to finish things, such as termination. While termination simply means to end the project or activity without any implication that a goal related to the matter has been reached, completion means that we (in some way) reach a goal for the project or activity. For example, we might terminate the race before we have run the full distance or we might complete the race by breaking the finishing tape. In this context it is completion rather than termination that is relevant, since death will automatically mean that all the projects and activities we are involved in will be terminated. Still, there are different ways to complete something.

To illustrate, the only way we can complete the race is by breaking the finishing tape, and what it is to complete the race is constitutive of the race. On the other hand, a sculpture might be completed in a number of different ways and it is the sculptor who decides when the work is completed. A thesis in philosophy is completed when we reach the goals that are a combination of generally agreed upon standards for a thesis in philosophy and our own goals for that thesis. Hence the criteria for whether something is completed or not might be purely subjective and up to ourselves to decide upon, or they might be intersubjectively decided upon or the result of a long social tradition or they might even be objective. Furthermore, what are considered as end-states or goals might change during the process or project.

Some projects might have end-states that cannot be reached under less than optimal conditions – for example, character development is generally thought to be a never-ending story since the ideal character is, indeed, ideal. Other projects might not have any proper end-states and could go on forever under optimal conditions – intimate personal relationships are often portrayed like that. Yet other projects do have or can be given end-states that can be reached (even if we might not reach them for different reasons), such as the project of writing a thesis in philosophy. Even if the end-state or goal we actually reach might be very different from the one we had in mind when we initiated the project. The last comment indicates that something can be completed according to one standard and still not be completed according to another standard.

Having this in mind, in what way could we complete the above-mentioned type of projects? The alternatives to completing them would seem to be either actively terminating them or just letting them go on without involving ourselves in either their continuation or ending until death terminates them. The latter two options would seem to coincide when we are the only ones involved in the project, or the only ones bringing the project forward.

Let us take a professional project we are involved in together with other people. One way to complete it would be to reach the overall goal of the project, but when we are dying time is likely to be too scarce for that. An alternative is that we reach a partial goal for the project or try to make sure that someone else brings it to completion. On the other hand, we might also actively terminate the project if we have the power to do so. Or we might just cease doing what we do in the project and allow it to continue without our involvement. More or less, we might fare similarly with the personal and societal projects we are involved in. However, when it comes to economic projects perhaps completion is more about transferring responsibility and the economic benefits to someone else rather than reaching a goal for these projects.

Having said something about what kind of worldly affairs we might complete and what it is to complete them, we can ask: why would that benefit us when dying?

Value to the dying person and others

From a well-being perspective, completing the projects we are involved with will often bring us satisfaction and hence raise our well-being. On the other hand, to complete the projects we are involved in will require both time and energy, which might be better used elsewhere in a way that will raise our well-being even more. In other words, the cost of completing the project might be too great to warrant the benefit. Hence, generally it might not be warranted to complete one's projects, especially considering that we might not actually be able to complete them fully but only complete them partially or hand them over to someone else for completion.

A further problem here might be the extent to which such a completion would emphasize our 'social death' (Sudnow 1967; Seale 1998; Lawton 2000). In the section on awareness of death we looked at an example from Lawton (2000) where a woman, Fiona, was reluctant to expose to her family that she was close to death since that would mean they would take over her projects or responsibilities in the family and emphasize her already marked social death. Similar reasons could be given for why we might be reluctant actively to complete or withdraw from projects we are involved in. On the other hand, it might be an essential part of our self-identity to be the kind of person who completes the projects we are involved in and hence mark that we are still the same person as before if we complete what we are involved in when we are about to die.

If we also consider the well-being benefits and costs to other people, we might have a *prima facie* moral reason to complete the projects that involve or affect these other people and where completion would make their lives better or where non-completion would worsen their lives. For example, if we do not sort out and complete our economic projects there might be a lot of conflict among our close ones after we are dead (of course, this might happen anyway but we will then have done what we can to avoid it). Hence, we might have moral reasons to complete our projects to the extent that they will bring benefits to other people, but also have moral reasons to abstain from completing our projects if it will be detrimental to other people or if time can be better spent. Returning to the woman in Lawton's account, it seems that the risk of her experiencing social death has to be weighed against the fact that her family needs to prepare for how to take care of her responsibilities and projects after she is gone. But, as indicated in the section on awareness, perhaps we can arrange the affairs of the dying person after she is dead without too much trouble and hence avoid emphasizing her social death.

Moving on to an objective list perspective, the most pertinent ideas in relation to the completion of projects are the ones about achievements and the ones about being a certain kind of person (indicated in the above comment on self-identity). To the extent that achievements are important to a good life, it would seem that achievements in which the goal of the achievement is fulfilled would add more than achievements where this is not the case. Perhaps not reaching any goal at all would actually disqualify the activity as an achievement. Hence, if we complete the thesis once started on, it will *ceteris paribus* add more to our lives than if we terminate the work on this thesis, given that termination does not result in even greater achievements being added to our lives. Supposedly different achievements will add differently to our lives and we have to distinguish between greater and smaller achievements when assessing how they add to our lives.

One important aspect of achievements affecting how they add to our lives is the effort put into the achievement on our behalf. This will enable us to achieve even if we are lacking in initial or predisposed qualifications, powers or abilities. Hence, for a physically impaired person, living on her own might be quite an achievement, which it is not for someone not thus impaired. On the other hand, if two people with the same initial qualifications and powers (acquired and others) engage in the same activity but with different outcomes, we might judge one of them a greater achievement than the other. Hence, the result of the achievement is also important to how it adds to our lives. Moreover, one of the things that make the result a greater achievement is how it adds to the lives of other people, i.e. whether the activity benefits other people or not. So it would seem we have at least three different criteria for whether an achievement adds to a life or not and for how much it adds: the effort put into the achievement, the result of this achievement and the value to people[3] (us and others) of this result.

Keeping this in mind, would the completion of wordly affairs at the end of life make for a better dying? If we do complete our affairs and they are not hurtful to other people (or even benefit them) it would seem to make our life somewhat better. Moreover, since we are dying (with weakening powers) it might take some effort and, hence, it might be quite an achievement. On the other hand, since we might not have time to complete them according to the original plan or the overall goal but only complete them partially or leave it over to others to bring them to completion, it might not add much extra to the achievement already made. That is, the greater part of the achievement that adds to our lives will already have been made and what we can complete is likely to be of minor importance to the value of our lives.

To take an example, let us say that I have worked the greater part of my life on a project to help homeless people. I want to complete my involvement in the project (since I am dying) by gathering all the knowledge and experience and ideas about it, together with all the paperwork, and leave it to those who are supposed to continue the project. Such a completion will add somewhat to achievement and ease, even if it is not essential to the continuation of the project. However, the greater part of the achievement adding to my life has already been made and hence the completion is likely to make little difference compared to that. Moreover, if this completion was essential to the continuation of the project we would have moral reasons to carry it out long before we were dying.

In conclusion, there is something to the idea that we will *ceteris paribus* benefit from completing our worldly affairs before we die, on any axiological account. However, this completion might not add very much to our lives and hence not be worth the time and effort it takes. Moreover, it might emphasize that we are no longer an active part of society or the social context we inhabit, i.e. voice that we are 'socially dead'. The strongest argument for completion is found in the moral responsibility we might have for completion, to the extent that completion will benefit other people (or when the lack of completion will hurt other people).

Normative aspects of a completed life

It is reasonable to leave the question of completion up to the individual patient and to enable those who want to complete their projects to do so. However, carers will have reason to make clear to the patient the extent to which his or her completion will benefit other people or not.

A possible problem here is the aspect of justice, i.e. if enabling a patient to complete his or her project is overly demanding in resources we might be hindered in enabling such a completion, especially since it would seem to emphasize the difference and prior inequality between patients, i.e. patients with a life full of projects (to many constitutive of a good life) would get a greater share of resources than a patient without such a life. Palliative care should not be expected to right the earlier injustices of society, but nor should it emphasize them.

End of life review

Another substantial preparation that, it is often argued, we should engage in at the end of life is to make a life review, or to: 'assess [our] lives for meaningfulness' (Momeyer 1988: 67). We need to say something about what it implies to make such a review or assessment before we move on to discuss whether that would add to the goodness of dying.[4]

Reviewing our life implies that we look back at our life and try to find that it has, or try to give it, certain features like value, point, meaning, direction, coherence. This is sometimes expressed as if we should be able to find a narrative or make a narrative about our life. Moreover, it is argued that we would benefit from *telling* the narrative of our life.[5] However, since I do not really find the narrative metaphor clarifying I will more or less avoid it henceforth.

It would seem that what we should find in life could be boiled down to the following essential features: value to myself, value to others, direction. We should also be able to understand why it went the way it did. A life will have direction to the extent that there is an overall goal (or goals) that the life moves towards. Let me make a few short comments about understanding before concentrating on the aspects of value and direction. Since understanding is something that would be the result of making a review, not something we would actually find in a life, and I might also understand a life without value and direction, the benefit of understanding would be intimately linked to the understanding in itself. However, even if understanding in itself can provide me with the well-being benefit of order or knowledge, I will boldly claim that the content of understanding is likely to affect our life even more; hence the reason for concentrating on value and direction.

Ideally, when I am making a life review, life should be found to have value to me and others and direction. It seems obvious that a life can have one without the other. Someone might live life with no overall goal or goals (not even to achieve value) and still, as it happens, add value to his and other persons' lives. On the other hand, someone might live life with an overall goal, even though the striving for and achievement of this goal does not add any value to his or other persons' lives. However, since it is far from clear what it takes for a life to have direction, let me elaborate somewhat on that before we take a look at the possible value of reviewing our lives when dying.

Regarding direction we need to distinguish between the conscious goals or direction we have strived towards and the goals or direction that can be attributed to our lives from the outside. In other words, trying to move in one direction with our life might not result in actually moving in that direction, or it might, from the outside, be interpreted as moving in another direction. For example, we might have as an overall goal in life to become a better person according to a fundamentalistic reading of the Bible, but from the outside it is interpreted as if we move away from becoming a better person and instead turn into a more moralistic and bigoted person. Or there might be a discrepancy because we are not successful in moving in the direction that we want to go. Or we might, in striving for a certain goal, also achieve other goals (not strived for), such as when we strive to become better golf players and at the same time achieve fame and fortune (however unimportant that is to us).

A problem here is what criteria a life should fulfil in order to have direction or a goal that it moves towards. In a sense it seems that even the most planless life could, at some level of abstraction, be fitted into a scheme of goals that gives it a certain direction. Hence, if moving beyond the conscious goals actually held by people in relation to their own lives, we risk making the idea of direction rather empty. Moreover, in this context, where finding direction in our lives is supposed to make for a better death, we might ask whether the important thing is our subjective view of what direction life has had or the objective or outside view of that direction.

I started out my life as a fundamentalist Christian, studied physics, philosophy and economics, then worked as a nurse's assistant and moved slowly away from my fundamentalist Christian beliefs to a rather liberal view. What is the direction of my life up to now – could we claim that all this has been a move in the direction of a philosophy doctorate, or that after a series of somewhat planless moves I ended up writing a thesis in philosophy?

The reason why both interpretations seem acceptable is that we might provide a number of different reasons for why we do the things we do, all plausible. It is, of course, difficult (especially in retrospect) to decide which of the reasons made us move in one direction rather than in another. Hence, we might claim that I had similar reasons for being a fundamentalist Christian and for starting to study philosophy, i.e. a serious interest in ideas and beliefs. Or we might claim that I started to study philosophy because I was unsatisfied with and unknowingly critical of the answers provided by my fundamentalist beliefs. We might also claim that I simply took an interest in philosophy without it being related in any way to my fundamentalist beliefs. We might perhaps find other plausible interpretations. Moreover, the reason why I started studying philosophy might not be the same reason why I have written a thesis in philosophy. That is, my life might have direction in that the different steps are related to each other but the starting point and the end result might not have very much to do with each other (except being related to me in some way). If the reason why I started doing philosophy was to find support for my fundamentalist beliefs that is not why I have written a thesis in philosophy. Of course, someone might claim that they are related in that I now try to question fundamentalist beliefs, but that only seems to prove my point about the difficulty of finding an objective direction in a life, i.e. the possibility of always providing alternative explanations. This should perhaps make us a bit suspicious about the existence of objective direction in a life or at least about our ability to get at it.

Value to the dying person and others

From the well-being perspective, it must be noted that the important aspect is whether I find my life to have had value and direction or accept the views of others on this. Hence, how my life might be viewed from the outside (except by myself in retrospect) or objectively will only be indirectly important.

Being the kind of persons we are it is likely to be important for most of us to find that our lives have had both value and direction and realizing that they have not might be devastating to our well-being (see Frankl 1963). That is, it might colour all our experiences to the degree that nothing might actually compensate for this blow. In Tolstoy's short story about Ivan Illych's death this is exactly where the protagonist ends up when he starts to review the life he thought successful and good. He finds that the things he has devoted his attention to – career, outward behaviour, others' opinions about him – are of no real value and he realizes that he has more or less wasted his life. Another way to express this might be to say that it is important to most people's self-identity that what they have done with their lives fits well into this identity (Lawton 2000), and it would be a considerable blow to find out that my self-identity is mistaken or does not fit well with what I have done with my life.

The question is then whether we should venture on such a dangerous journey when we might arrive at an answer that will actually lower our well-being. Perhaps it is often better to live with the unfounded opinion (if having such an opinion) that our lives have had value and direction and not delve into this and find that they really have not. Even accepting the idea that it is possible to find some direction in any life, we might not find the kind of direction or value that will satisfy us. It would seem that a desperate attempt to find some value and direction in a life emphasizes the lack of these.

Feigenberg (1979), presenting a psychotherapeutic method for the dying person, claims that the therapist should try to value the person for what she has done with her life, even if the dying person sees it as a failure (see also Beck-Friis 1990). However, it is not clear whether there is a truth or sincerity condition attached to this; that is, whether one is allowed to rearrange the facts so as to end up with a life that has had value and direction, even if the therapist does not really find this.

A similar argument could be given from a desire fulfilment approach, with the exception that, in such an approach, being in bad faith will not actually benefit you, since it is only actual desire fulfilment that makes a life valuable. So, in such an approach we do not risk anything of value in exploring whether our life has had value and direction. But we might still end up with the conclusion that it did not have the value and direction we wanted it to have.

From an objective list standpoint it seems obvious that if a life contains value to me and others, it is a better life, the idea about relationships supporting the idea about being valuable to other people. However, it is less clear why direction would, on any of the suggested items, make for a better dying. One idea could be that it is instrumental in relation to achievements, but then it is the achievements that are important, not that our lives have been directed in relation to these achievements.

To illustrate, if the important achievement adding to my life is the writing of a thesis in philosophy (perhaps doubted by the majority), this achievement would not seem lesser if I ended up writing it after planlessly moving around than if the whole of my foregoing life was a preparation for it. Of course, this preparation might have been necessary and without it I would not have written the thesis, but that does not change the fact that the achievement was the thesis, not its preparations. That is, the preparations without the thesis would not have added to my life (if they do not contain achievements or other valuables in their own right). Hence, our lives might need direction towards goals to achieve these goals, but it is the achievement not the direction that adds to our lives here. Perhaps it should be added, however, that if these preparations were not necessary to achieve the goals in question I could have put my time to better use by achieving other things instead of just planlessly moving about. However, that would not necessarily have added to the direction of my life. In other words, these achievements might have been totally unrelated to one another.

Another idea is that the importance of direction has to do with self-determination. That is, a life in which there is direction must be directed by someone (or something) and if our life has had direction it might be a sign of us having been self-determined and having directed our lives, not just been moved along by whatever or whoever came in our way. However, since the direction of a life might be the result of going with the flow or being directed by someone or something else, this will presuppose that the direction can be attributed to us and our decisions and goals in some way. To be sure, here the important thing is that we have been self-determined, not that we have a sense of being or having been self-determined.

Following the above discussion, even if every step we have taken has been the result of deciding in accordance with what we want, this might not imply that our lives have had overall direction. In other words, we might not have wanted to take steps directed at one and the same goal all through life; instead we might have followed different wants at different times or our wants may have changed during our lives.

Hence, when I started studying philosophy I made a self-determined decision, but even if my philosophy studies were part of the reason why I lost my fundamentalist beliefs, I did not choose to lose them. That is, the steps that took me from evening classes in philosophy to the loss of my fundamentalist beliefs were not steps directed by me in the same direction. Furthermore, had I known at the time that my philosophy studies would have ended up in me losing my beliefs, I would have been more reluctant to pursue them. That is, if I had full knowledge about what they would result in, I would not (at the time) have wanted to engage in them. Then my life would (possibly) still have been directed in line with my fundamentalist beliefs and have had an overall direction, something I am glad it has not. This also indicates that if we want to pursue our life with an overall direction, we might need to be omniscient in order not to risk losing this direction.

Following this, it would seem easier to attribute the direction to God or fate or something along those lines, indicating that our lives are given value in being used for some higher purpose or by being directed by something outside our control. Now, if we are directed by something outside our control we might perhaps be thankful if this brings us the things that add value to our lives, but it will do so at the price of self-determination. Moreover, the value added is in these things rather than in what brought them to us. Hence, if we achieve things because we are brought to the point where we can achieve by God or by our own efforts we can still claim that it is the achievement that adds to our life. However, if we partly owe this achievement to something outside of us, it would seem to lessen the value this achievement brings to our lives. If, on the other hand, our achievements are made even greater because they are made with a guide who has full knowledge at hand, the lesser effort of ours might perhaps be compensated by the greater and more valuable result of that achievement. To write a thesis with the guidance of a tutor would seem a somewhat lesser achievement than writing it all on your own. On the other hand, if this results in a greater achievement or the thesis would not have been written without the tutor's help it is better that the tutor intervenes. Still, it is the achievement that brings value to my life, not the direction.

Is there another aspect of this that brings value to my life, i.e. that we are important to some higher power and this will add value to our lives? First, that our lives have direction is only an indication of that. To be sure, our lives could have had value to this higher power without us being used or directed in this way. Furthermore, when we picture valuable relationships to ourselves, being directed or used by the other party would seem to lessen the value of such relationships rather than enhance the value of them. Arguably, when someone uses us for their purposes, even if we admit the value of that purpose, we often think that it is less beneficial to the value of our lives than if we were not used thus. This is the basic idea in one of the formulations of Kant's categorical imperative – that we should treat human beings always as goals in themselves and not only as means to our own goals.

In conclusion, that our lives have direction might be instrumental in adding achievements to our lives. However, I have found no reason to think that direction, in itself, adds anything to our lives apart from the satisfaction that might be associated with this or the desire that we have for our lives to have direction. Regarding telling the narrative of one's life I think it can be said that this is likely to bring value to a life in much the same way as being present at someone's death bed will bring value. That is, there is supposedly a great satisfaction in telling the story of one's life and even if it has not been a success it implies that someone is willing to take time and interest in us and our lives. Something, I take it, will raise the well-being of almost anyone. However, it must be remembered that it can also be painful to tell someone else about a failed and wasted life, realizing and admitting that life had neither much in terms of direction nor value (compare the comments on expressivism in the section on self-control in Chapter 4).

> Normative aspects of a reviewed life
>
> Being a consequentialist, I have no principled problem with lying. However, since lying will often lead to worse consequences in the long run it seems that we generally have reasons to abstain from it. In this case, even if the patient's well-being would be benefited from being wrongly convinced about direction and value in life, I think we should be careful not to try to convince the patient of this in face of obvious evidence to the contrary. However, we have reasons to try to focus on the good parts of a patient's life and we should not, in my mind, rob the patient of a false belief about this – unless the patient expressedly wants to have true beliefs about his or her life. On the other hand, professional carers have strong reasons to take time to listen to patients telling about their lives, whether good or bad, since this implies taking an interest in the patient at hand.

Staging one's departure

The *Ars Moriendi* tradition emphasized the staging of one's own departure as one of the important things for receiving a good death (see Ariés 1974, 1981). Indeed, the death bed was viewed much as a stage where the main character, i.e. the dying person, was to be surrounded by the important characters of his life. Ariés (1981: 19) expresses this in the following way: '[the dying person] presided, as was the custom, over the ceremony of her own death'. We find something similar in Callahan (1993: 11): 'The visitors chatted and gossiped, as if it were just another social gathering of the kind she [Callahan's grandmother] had presided over for years.' In the following quotation from Kübler-Ross (1969: 5) we see something similar in the dying person arranging his affairs and saying goodbye.

I remember as a child the death of a farmer. He fell from a tree and was not expected to live. He asked simply to die at home, a wish that was granted without questioning. He called his daughters into the bedroom and spoke with each of them alone for a few minutes. He arranged his affairs quietly, though he was in great pain, and distributed his belongings and his land, none of which was to be split until his wife should follow him in death. He also asked each of his children to share in the work, duties, and tasks that he had carried on until the time of the accident. He asked his friends to visit him once more, to bid good-bye to them. Although I was a small child at the time, he did not exclude me or my siblings. We were allowed to share in the preparations of the family just as we were permitted to grieve with them until he died.

According to Walter (1994) this is part and parcel of the modern idea of a good death, as is voiced in the following quotation from Levine, which he cites (with the comment that it was supposed to be a caricature of this idea about a good death):

> When we think of our death, we imagine ourselves surrounded by loving friends, the room filled with quietude that comes from nothing more to say, all business finished; our eyes shining with love and with a whisper of profound wisdom as to the transiency of life, we settle back into the pillow, the last breath escaping like a vast 'Ahh!' as we depart gently into the light.
>
> (Walter 1994: 60)

Value to the dying person and others

From a well-being approach the staging of one's own departure would seem to find some support. That is, a lot of people (perhaps even most people) generally enjoy and desire to be the centre of other people's attention and to decide how to have things; at least, being the centre of the attention of people they appreciate or are closely related to. However, at the end of life when we are weakened by disease, when beauty does not come from within but has stayed within, when we might be disfigured and smelly (see Lawton 2000 for a vivid description of dying people's bodily decay), other people's attention might be disturbing rather than a cause for enjoyment. For the same reasons we might not bother much about calling the shots or staging and presiding over our departure. Moreover, to stage one's departure in the rather patriarchial way portrayed in the quotation from Kübler-Ross – arranging affairs, distribute belongings, passing on the torch of carrying out what the dying person has begun or uttering words of wisdom – implies that we have affairs, belongings, important projects and wisdom and also a special standing in the group of close ones. Just imagine the farmer's maid or farmhand in the same situation. What would they have to arrange or distribute? In effect, this might not be applicable to a large number of dying people in society today, especially given that most people die at an age when they have already lost much of this.

To the extent that we have affairs to arrange or belongings to distribute, we might of course have moral reasons to do so. However, if we have a moral reason to do so we should not wait until our death bed to sort out these things since that would jeopardize them being done at all. That is, there are no guarantees that we can do what is morally required of us on our death bed.

We might stage our death in a less patriarchial manner than the one portrayed above. That is, we might draw on the quotation from Callahan and make it into a social gathering of our liking – whether it is a quiet dinner with our closest friends or a boisterous party with the people we have been used to having a ball with. To the extent that we are not bothered by the above-mentioned problems, this is likely to be beneficial in relation to our well-being. Dying people might not be in a state in which they are able to stage or benefit from staging their departure. Besides describing the bodily decay in dying people, Lawton (2000) describes the loss of self in terms of loss of important relationships, i.e. social death, before people actually physically die. Hence, this form of staging is not open to everyone and it might actually be open to very few dying people.

Normative aspects of a staged departure

If the dying person wants to stage her death in a specific way, carers should enable her to do so, provided it is reasonable given the claims of justice. As indicated above, staging might be open mainly for those people who are already well off in different ways, and carers should not provide these people with even more resources to the cost of other, less benefited, patients. That is, a person with greater social resources might be more motivated to stage his or her departure, a staging that might demand resources from the palliative carers, and we should be careful about giving extra resources to people just because they are able to come up with and express desires about how they want life to be.

However, having this justice claim concerning resources in mind, palliative care cannot be the place where every inequality due to the life the dying patient has lived is balanced and, given this restriction, we should enable staging to the extent that it is important to the dying person.

Conclusions and relevance to palliative care

In this chapter we have discussed whether we should prepare for death in any specific way to enable a good dying and death. We have discussed whether we have reasons to prepare in a ritualistic way, whether we have reasons to complete our worldly affairs, whether we have reasons to make an end of life review and, finally, whether we have reasons to stage our departure in a specific way.

In relation to rituals we distinguished between rituals and formulas, where the former were implied to have a symbolic meaning beyond the actual actions we do and the latter are just a way to order a set of actions. We found that rituals had ambiguous support, and to a large extent the benefits of rituals were dependent on them being well known to us. Hence, we found it problematic to establish new rituals when the old ones seem to have been 'worn out'. However, it was also argued that formulas for how to prepare or act in the face of death might to some extent be a replacement for rituals, retaining a large part of the benefits of rituals – with less risk of being repressive or empty, since they do not make any symbolic claims. In both cases it was argued that rituals and formulas might hinder a more spontaneous manner of facing or dealing with death. This is relevant to palliative care, since it has been argued that palliative care should help to establish new rituals in the face of death and we need to discuss whether this would actually benefit dying people or not, and whether it would be possible to establish such rituals or whether we can find any substitutes that do much of the task.

In relation to the completion of worldly affairs it was argued that our completion might not make much difference to how the projects we have add to our lives, since we will seldom be able to reach the overall goal of the project when dying, due to lack of strength and time. If anything we might have a moral reason to complete a project, to the extent that such a completion will ease the lives of other people, or not completing the project will cause other people serious trouble, i.e. small inconveniences should not be reason enough. This will be relevant to palliative care to the extent that people want to be enabled to complete the projects they are involved in; and to the extent that this is important to people, regardless of whether they actually have strong reasons for this or not, I see no principled reason why we could not help dying people with this, at least to the extent it does not take resources from more important aspects and does not hinder us from providing other dying people in our care with as good a death as possible.

In relation to the making of an end of life review it was argued that even if it might be satisfying to look back at a good life, it might also be problematic to look back at a not so good life, and hence it will not be generally good for all dying people to make such a review. This was supported by the fact that we did not find any good reasons to support the view that life having direction (apart from the value it has had) should be of value as such. The relevance to palliative care has to do with the fact that we sometimes find the idea that life should be reviewed at the end and again we need to discuss such an idea critically. What we found to have support was that carers and others should take time to listen to the dying patient who wants to tell about his or her life, which in general could be viewed as support for the idea that palliative carers should care for the dying patient in whatever way the dying patient finds comforting. Moreover, since telling about oneself and one's life is an important part of any social intercourse, listening to a patient's story is a way to postpone the social death of the patient.

In relation to the staging of one's departure, it was argued that staging in the more patriarchial manner was mainly open for a limited number of people (i.e. patriarchs) and hence of limited interest to a good death. On the other hand, enabling people to stage or fashion death as they see fit, whatever that implies, will be beneficial to most people. The problem is that most people might not be in the condition to do much staging when death approaches, as both the literature on dying people and my own experience with them witness. To the extent that palliative care should enable the dying patient to die as good a death as possible, and staging is important to the dying patient, this should of course be enabled as long as such a staging does not rob the other patients of resources.

In effect, the rather uncontroversial conclusion of this chapter is that the preparations could in some cases add to the good death of a dying person but we could in other cases do as well without them. Hence, we do not find strong reasons to take a definite stand when it comes to these preparations when caring for dying persons.

Notes

1 See Callahan (1993) and Clark and Seymour (1999).
2 See, for example Glaser and Strauss (1965: 103, 127), Dunstan (1978) and Saunders and Baines (1983).
3 Or, even more generally, creatures that can benefit or suffer (in a wider interpretation than the hedonistic one) from our actions. For example, it would seem quite an achievement to save an endangered species.
4 We find this idea in different versions in, for example, Glaser and Strauss (1965), Feigenberg (1977, 1979), Lindqvist (1980), Larsson (1984), Ternestedt (1994, 1998), Lantz (1992) and Nuland (1993).
5 See Lantz (1992), de Marinis (1998), Clark and Seymour (1999) and Janssens (2001).

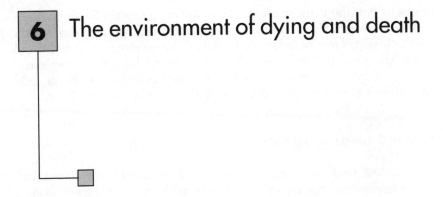

6 The environment of dying and death

This chapter deals with the environment of dying and death and what should characterize such an environment, including things like peacefulness, the presence of other people and the presence of technology.

A peaceful death

Daniel Callahan (1993) labels the combination of different characteristics of good death he presents a peaceful death. However, here I will discuss whether a peaceful death in its own right is generally good for us or not. The idea about a peaceful death is also something that is recurrently found in the palliative literature.[1] In Walter's (1994: 109) words: 'In some British hospices, staff are acutely aware of how nice and middle-class they are and how they want patients to die peacefully.'

First, we might distinguish between situations and people being peaceful or between *external* and *internal peacefulness*. External peacefulness implies an environment that is quiet rather than noisy, calm rather than busy, harmonious rather than chaotic or distorted, perhaps also beautiful rather than ugly; perhaps serenity would describe such a situation well. A traditional example of this (also used metaphorically in relation to peace and peacefulness) is heaven. Internal peacefulness, on the other hand, implies calmness of mind, restfulness, lack of internal conflicts or conflicts with the environment, lack of aggravation and perhaps also being morally satisfied or undisturbed by the way one leads one's life. First it must be pointed out that even if external peacefulness might be necessary in some cases to achieve internal peacefulness, it seems possible to be internally peaceful even in an externally non-peaceful environment. Martyrs have often been portrayed as internally peaceful in the midst of torture and other terrible situations. Even in less idealized circumstances we sometimes meet people who remain internally peaceful in situations that would make most of us aggravated and upset. Moreover, people might lack internal peacefulness even in an externally peaceful environment. Hence, internal peacefulness is logically independent of external peacefulness even if not always empirically so.

Value to the dying person and others

From a hedonistic perspective an externally peaceful environment will probably often increase our well-being and it might even be the case that most people appreciate a peaceful environment when dying, especially since they might be more sensitive to noise and chaos due to their disease. However, it is not difficult to imagine someone finding such an enviroment boring and being more appreciative of an environment that is noisy, busy and chaotic; that is, an environment that they do not consider to be a forecourt to eternal rest (Walter 1994).

Generally, an argument against dying at specific palliative institutions is that the environment has too many of the above features. Some people do not want to experience deprivation of their busy and intense life before death, due to the boredom associated with such deprivation. However, it might not only be the boredom that is problematic; a more serious problem is if the dying person interprets the external peacefulness around her as if she is already socially dead (Lawton 2000). Lawton finds that people with different class backgrounds seem to have somewhat different ideas on the extent to which they want their environment to be externally peaceful or not, at least to the extent of wanting to be placed in a single-bed room or a room with more than one bed. Hence, ideas on peacefulness are obviously related to the kind of life one appreciates, which in turn can be related to things like class.

If we look at external peacefulness from the objective list perspective, could it be good for me to be in an externally peaceful environment even if it does not cause a rise in my well-being or it causes a lowering of that well-being? Personally I find it difficult to see any plausible reasons why it would be so. A possible reason is that an externally peaceful environment is the kind of environment that best expresses respect for the dying person (this has to some extent been discussed in the section on dignity).

However, imagine someone from a milieu where people are expected to gather around the dying person expressing grief, mourning and lamentations in a loud way (see, for example, Saunders and Barnes 1983). For example, the following description is from a Swedish author describing his juvenile years as the son of a missionary man in Congo: 'grief is a demon to be exorcised from the body. You scream and cry until all powers and emotions are drained' (Hagerfors 2003: 178, my translation). Coming from such a milieu, this way to express grief is presumably the best way to show the dying person respect and the best way to acknowledge his importance. Now, if someone with such a background were to die in an externally peaceful environment this could be interpreted by him as if he has no one (from his social milieu) to whom he matters, or in other words emphasize his 'social death'. External peacefulness is not bad *per se* for him, but an indication of something that is bad for him (and would probably also have a negative effect on his well-being). Hence, it is obvious that external peacefulness is not the only way of showing the dying person respect. Moreover, even if solemnity and external peacefulness are the traditional way of showing respect in our culture some people might be more interested in disrespect at the end of life, due to the above problems with external peacefulness. In other words, we might show such people more respect by letting the environment they die in be busy and lively. Here it is important to be wary of the ease with which we relate to people from other cultures in a stereotyped manner. In a study of Swedish palliative carers it was found that carers view uncharacteristic wants or behaviour by people with a Swedish background as individual variations, but uncharacteristic wants or behaviour by people with a foreign background as culturally dependent.[2] We should not take for granted that coming from a certain culture implies something specific about whether one appreciates an externally peaceful environment or not. We should try to find out how this particular person wants her dying environment to be.

In conclusion, even if external peacefulness might often be considered a proper feature of the environment in which to care for dying people, this would depend on what the dying person appreciates, which in turn might depend on the kind of milieu she has been used to. Hence, it cannot be claimed that an externally peaceful environment is universally conducive of a good or better death for all people or the best way to show respect for people. On the other hand, when people are affected by disease they will often be more sensitive to noise and chaos and there might in many cases be hedonistic reasons to keep the external environment peaceful. This obviously does not apply to all dying people, and certainly not to people in all the different stages of dying.

Normative aspects of a peaceful death

As before, carers should be sensitive to what the dying patient appreciates concerning a peaceful environment. However, since different patients may want different things and the less peaceful environment some patients might want is problematic for other patients, it is necessary to strike a balance between peace and its alternatives. Still, it is important for carers not to presuppose that dying persons automatically want an externally peaceful environment, or its opposite.[3]

A public death

One important feature of the tame death found in the writings of Philippe Ariés is the idea about death being public:

> the vile and ugly death of the Middle Ages, is . . . the secret death that is without witness or ceremony: the death of the traveler on the road, or the man who drowns in the river, or the stranger whose body is found at the edge of a field, or even the neighbor who is struck down for no reason . . . The dying person must be the center of a group of people.
>
> (Ariés 1981: 11, 18)

The ideal was a death where people were gathered at the dying person's death bed. In modern palliative literature and literature about good death we still find the ideal of not dying alone, as was seen in the quotation from Walter (1994) in the section in Chapter 5 on staging one's departure.[4] Today it is, however, expected that we should have our close ones present or, if that is not possible, someone from the care personnel. The idea about all and sundry attending our death has been lost.

It might be argued that the publicity of ancient deaths might have been more or less unavoidable due to the more crowded and close contact of everday life.[5] That is, there was simply no room for dying alone. Hence, Ariés might be making a virtue out of necessity when advocating a public death. Still, let us treat his idea as a serious suggestion for what makes for a good death. Pursuing this thought, it seems that there are two different reasons to die a public death. First, it would seem to acknowledge the dying person to have been (or still to be) an important part of a certain community – be it society or family or the group of close ones. Second, it precludes the dying person from being alone in dying.

Traditionally the death of a person would have been attended by a number of different people, all there to acknowledge the importance of the dying person: close ones, people living in the vicinity, perhaps representatives from the community and unknown people who just happened to pass by. Drawing on this aspect of publicity, they would have been there as an act of social recognition, of acknowledging the dying person as playing or having played a social role in the community they represented, i.e. the community of close ones and family, of neighbours, of the village or town and perhaps even the human community. If people not personally affected by the person's death took the time and effort to attend his death bed, this would have implied that his death was an important event even outside his very inner circles and that he was a recognized part of the community they represented. Is it indeed such a confirmation and, if so, in what way might such confirmations add to the goodness of our death? Here it must be noted that the distinction between who belongs to our close ones and who does not might not be all that clear. For example, of the general public that might attend our death some will be totally unknown to us, some we will know by reputation, some we will know personally even if they are not close. However, in this context I will take it to be clear enough to enable a separate discussion of these different people.

The second aspect of a public death is simply that it might be problematic to be alone in dying and death. To have someone present at the death bed is something that the literature almost universally seem to view as the ideal way to die. For example, in the Swedish Parliamentary Commission Report on Palliative Care it is claimed that 'patients should not have to die alone' (SOU 2001: my translation). In Elias (1985) the problem of loneliness in (modern) dying is discussed at length.

Value to the dying person and others

Let us start with the aspect of not being alone in dying and death. Obviously, many (most) of us enjoy and desire the company of others; especially the company of close ones and especially in situations of trouble and distress. Hence, from a hedonistic and desire fulfilment approach to value we are likely to find strong support for not dying alone. However, this picture needs to be balanced: first, as to the reasons we might have for dying alone; second, as to which company would actually benefit us (or benefit us the most).

If my close ones are distressed by seeing me die, it might not be beneficial for me (or them) to have them present at my death bed. Moreover, if there is an unresolved conflict between us that causes aggravation, I will probably not be benefited by having them there. However, I might have more positive reasons for not wanting them there – for example, that I want them to remember me as I used to be and look before disease took the best of me. Furthermore, there is some evidence that dying patients die when they are left alone, indicating that they might have trouble letting go if constantly in the company of someone, especially if in the company of someone close (Rinell-Hermansson 1990). Hence, if this prolongation is of no use to the dying person, we might have a reason to leave a dying person alone to enable him or her to die. Yet another reason why we might prefer to die alone is that we consider the time we have left too important to spend on other people and something we want to have to ourselves. As Weisman (1972: 40) claims, 'Some patients prefer solitude toward the end in order to collect their thoughts. Others, more gregarious, need family and friends.' If these are relevant reasons for being worse off having close ones present, would we still be better off having someone else present instead of dying alone?

To some extent it might be a better alternative, since someone not personally involved with me might be better suited to bring comfort and ease my anguish and I might also be less bothered about showing them my present condition. On the other hand, if I do not have any close ones or do not have any close ones that do show up, it might be more painful to be reminded that the only alternative to dying alone is to have someone not close attending my death bed. If so, I might actually prefer to die alone.

Moreover, if it is important that we do matter to other people (as most people would think), then to die only attended by someone who is paid to do it or who does not do it because *we* matter to them (i.e. they could have attended someone else's death bed instead) would seem to indicate that we do not really matter to other people in a relevant sense (or at least that we do not matter any more). Elias (1985) claims that we might be as lonely with people for whom we are not significant as when we are by ourselves. Generally, however, even someone who attends our death bed as part of their professional duties might take a personal interest in us and if so we would at least matter somewhat to them. So, having someone not close at our bedside will, in most cases, not worsen the situation – unless we positively prefer dying alone.

Apart from these hedonistic and desire fulfilment reasons for not dying alone, could it be argued from the idea about intimate personal relationships that we have reasons not to die alone? In an intimate personal relationship it would seem essential that we should spend time with a partner who is experiencing a troublesome situation. Presumably, it is one of the characterizing features of such a relationship and to the extent that close ones do not show up because they do not feel up to it, or do not want to miss the concert they have tickets for, we should probably question the intimacy of the relationship.

So, spending time together at the end of life will presumably add somewhat to the value of the intimate personal relationship. It might of course be asked whether it is more important to spend time at that time than at other times. Normally, we might choose not to spend time together knowing (or expecting) that we will spend time together at a later time, but that is not an option at the end of life when death might be expected at any time. Hence if spending time together in intimate personal relationships is one of the more valuable items on the objective list we should probably fill our last flickering moments with that.

On the other hand, if close ones do not attend the death bed because they they cannot stand to see their loved one in this state or cannot handle the situation well, this would seem to indicate the emotional closeness of the relationship. Perhaps it could be argued that such a relationship could have been better, since an ideal intimate personal relationship implies a willingness to pay the cost of comforting and supporting a troubled partner. However, we seldom live in ideal relationships and what happens at my death bed will not change the value of the relationships we have had to any significant degree. That is whether our close ones show up or not does not make that much difference to the value of the intimate personal relationship from the objective list perspective.

In conclusion, in the hedonistic and desire fulfilment approaches we find strong support for not dying alone, even if we also found some relevant reasons for not wanting to have anyone present at the death bed. In the objective list approach the support was more indirect, implying that an intimate personal relationship is likely to end up with close ones wanting to attend the death bed. But to the extent that we are close to someone we might be too distressed by the situation to be able to see the close one die. Moreover, since we do not live in ideal relationships, the distress might also cause conflicts and other troubles, making it better for the dying person to die alone.

What about the aspect of acknowledgement? Generally, to be acknowledged to be important to other people is likely to be something all of us (or almost all of us) desire and enjoy and something that is important for our image of ourselves as persons (Lawton 2000). Hence, if someone with whom we have been close shows up at our death bed and explicitly or implicitly expresses an acknowledgement of our importance to them, it is likely to bring about a better death for most of us. A difference between the two value approaches of hedonism and desire fulfilment is that with hedonism it is enough that we believe that we have been important even if we have not, since all that matters is how our well-being is affected, whereas with desire fulfilment, if we desire to be important and be acknowledged for this, it is only actual importance and recognition of such importance that will be beneficial to us.

From the objective list perspective, it would seem obvious that the idea about intimate personal relationships would give support to close ones attending the death bed and acknowledging the importance of their dying close one. In other words, people with whom we have had intimate and personal relationships are often likely to want to spend those last few hours of our lives with us and we are often likely to want to have them there.

However, disregarding well-being and desires, if the close ones were not present would that in any way reduce the value of their intimate personal relationship to the dying person? The value of the relationship will depend on the character of this relationship, and it seems obvious that intimate personal relationships can add more or less to our lives. Hence all intimate personal relationships have a certain character (synchronically and diachronically) and add a certain value to our life. Now, what will change the character of a relationship might be difficult to pinpoint – but obviously a relationship can change over time. What used to be an emotionally close and honest relationship can turn into a distant relationship in which we become secretive to one another. However, to distance oneself on one occasion or have a few secrets might not affect the relationship at all or if so only marginally. Consequently, being present at the death bed would not seem to be essential to the character of the relationship. Hence, from an objective list approach it does not seem to make much difference to the value of the relationship but it might of course reveal the true nature of this relationship (with the hedonistic cost following that).

In conclusion, from the perspective of acknowledgement we have reasons, in any axiological approach, to have our close ones spend time at our death bed. Moreover, they are likely to do so to the extent that they are close to us.

Could it be argued that we have similar reasons to have other people present at our death beds? From a hedonistic and desire fulfilment perspective it is obvious that we might benefit from being acknowledged as important within a wider social perspective – the neighbourhood, the village or town and perhaps even the human community. However, given the more individualized society we live in, where we are likely to value recognizable individual contributions more than anonymous collective contributions, it would seem that we should be recognized for the contribution *we* have made to the community in question. At least, such a specific recognition would presumably be more beneficial to us than a more general one from these two axiological approaches. The problem is that we do not all make recognizable contributions and some of us do not contribute at all to the community of which we are members.

Moving on to the objective list approach, would a public death add to the value of death and dying apart from any effects such a death will have on the well-being or desire fulfilment of the dying person? In the section on value it was suggested that achievements (i.e. social achievements or achievements important to society) were a possible item on such an objective list and that therefore we might imagine finding support for a public death from such a feature.

However, our social achievements do not seem to be greater *per se* for the acknowledgement we get for them. Obviously, in some cases, achievements need to be acknowledged in order to be achievements at all (for example, to be the most well known politician in a society) or, more importantly, if being acknowledged will make it easier for us to make achievements. We might nevertheless take part in society and achieve great things without getting any credit for this, and these things will not be made greater if we are acknowledged for achieving them. Hence, having a representative of the community at our bedside when we are about to die will not generally add anything to the achievements we have made within this community. It will just be a confirmation that we have made such achievements.

In conclusion, there are obviously hedonistic and desire fulfilment benefits in being acknowledged as individually important – from the more intimate social context as well as the more general social context. From an objective list perspective it is not as obvious why we would be better off for being acknowledged; it is instead something that follows from being involved in different types of relationships and something that we deserve when we have contributed to the social context in question. However, this would also imply that the death of someone who has not played an important social role might be worsened, since such a death will be markedly non-public in the sense relevant here. On the other hand, if publicity is made into the general norm for all deaths we would seem to lose much of the benefit, since it will no longer be the individual contribution of the person to the community that will be the reason why people attend his or her death bed.

Normative aspects of an acknowledged death

Carers should enable the patient's close ones to be present to the extent she so wishes. However, since there are also relevant reasons for wanting to be alone in death, they should be careful to respect such a wish. Here it is important to be clear about why the patient wants to be alone. Is it that she thinks no one is really botherered about her death and she does not want her desire for company to be frustrated once again, or is it a well thought through wish to actually die alone?

Even if the company of a professional carer at the end of life is sometimes viewed as an absolute norm, we should be careful not to make this into an excuse for not giving the patient company at other times. That is, even if she 'did at least not have to die alone' it might be poor consolation and it seems more or at least as important to spend time with the patient at other times.

A non-technological death

In Callahan we find the following claims:

Some will think that any life under any condition is better than no life at all, and such a position only feeds slavery to a technology that can always keep a body going just a bit longer . . . It should also be a death marked by consciousness, by a self-awareness that one is dying, that the end has come – but, even more pointedly, a death marked by self-possession, by a sense *that one is ending one's days awake, alert, and physically independent, not as a machine-sustained body or a body that has long ago lost its mind and self-awareness.*

(Callahan 1993: 180, 54, emphasis added)

In Kübler-Ross we find a similar reluctance about life-prolonging technology:

Dying becomes lonely and impersonal because the patient is often taken out of his familiar environment and rushed to an emergency room . . . He may cry for rest, peace and dignity, but he will get infusions, transfusions, a heart machine, or tracheotomy if necessary.

(Kübler-Ross 1969: 8)[6]

Traditionally, there has been some reluctance to use technology within palliative care,[7] even if there has been a change in how technology is viewed within this care.[8] This development has, however, resulted in a discussion about the medicalization of palliative care.[9]

Technological measures (henceforth also 'machines') are considered problematic to a good death in two ways. First, they might prolong a life in a way that will result in a bad (or worse) death. Second, they might make the context of death into something that precludes a good death (or makes for a worse death). For example, a death surrounded by machines might make it less familiar, less home-like, less beautiful, less independent or less natural. People might also, as a result of technology, focus on the wrong things in death. Let me start by saying something about the relation between technology and prolongation of life.

Prolonging life with technology

Following the discussion of the value of the event of death, it can be argued that as a general rule life should only be prolonged to the point where further life will not, on the whole, add positive value. In other words, the emphasis is on the deprivation factor, which implies that life should not be prolonged beyond the point where further life will be bad for us. However, the extinction factor gives us some reason to prolong even beyond this point in time if life is neutral, in order to postpone the time when we are all over.

Callahan argues that following some equivalent of the D-factor will lead us into something he calls 'technological brinkmanship', which is another word for attempts to try to move as close as possible to the line between worthwhile and non-worthwhile life using machines. In the wake of technological brinkmanship he sees two main problems: (a) the risk of overstepping the above line, since we do not 'understand technology well enough to know when and how in the course of dying to find medically the just-right moment to halt it' (Callahan 1993: 37); (b) the risk of making the context of death into something that does not make for a good death.

When we did not have technology helping us to prolong life, people died after just a short period of illness and did not end up in long periods of coma or unconsciousness before they died. Moreover, to the extent that people recovered, they did not have to suffer lingering disability: 'In the absence of effective medical treatment, it was left to the body to do its own unaided recovery. If it could do so, it did so rapidly. If it could not, death would come quickly' (Callahan 1993: 43). Callahan admits that:

> It does not pay attention to the pain that marked many earlier deaths, unrelieved by narcotics or analgesics. There were no respirators to relieve the suffocation induced by collapsing lungs, or drugs to control the erratic beat of a heart out of control, or antibiotics to stem gangrene or the torture of spreading bedsores. If the course of death was usually shorter, it could be and often was more intense in its agonies.
>
> (*Ibid.*: 52)

Still, what technology has brought us, together with longer lives, is also 'worse health, longer illnesses and slower deaths, longer aging and increased dementia' (*ibid.*: 47).[10] Hence, in using technology to push the limits of life further and further we will get even longer lives, but also worsening health, longer illnesses, slower deaths, longer ageing and increased dementia. These longer lives are not worth the price or, at least, since Callahan admits that the gain brought to us by medicine and technology is of a sort not easily wished away, technological brinkmanship takes this prolongation too far. Here, it is important to distinguish between different forms of technology. In Seymour *et al.* (2002) we find a study showing older participants to be reluctant to use technology to prolong life when close to death but, on the other hand, welcoming the use of technology to alleviate problematic symptoms. Still, even if we cannot generally avoid using technology to prolong our lives, at what point should we stop using it?

Callahan's argument implies that technology to prolong lives should not be used beyond the point where it will be instrumental to a good life (or death). In other words, it should be abated when it no longer results in worthwhile life for the person in question. Hence, the problem with technological brinkmanship does not seem to be that doctors try to follow what is implied by the D-factor, but that they interpret worthwhile life as coextensive with biological life and thus prolong the lives of the patients beyond this point:

> a stretching to the limit and beyond the power of technology to extend the life of organ systems independent of the welfare of the persons to whom they belong . . . The process of dying is also deformed when

there is an extended period of loss of consciousness well before we are actually dead. It is deformed when there is an exceedingly and unduly long period of debility and frailty before death. It is deformed when there is a lengthy period of pain and suffering prior to death ... we human beings have generated our own miseries when we allow technology to create a situation that produces exceedingly long periods of those evils.

(Callahan 1993: 41, 193)

That is, if doctors really put emphasis on the idea about worthwhile life they would have to take into account the effect of technology on the dying patient's life. Whether this makes for a better death or not will depend on the particular case at hand. So the main problem does not seem to be that technology runs amok but that the idea about sanctity of (biological) life has too strong a hold on physicians. The D-factor would probably have given us reason not to use technology to prolong life in the above cases. Still, I am not thereby implying that such a judgement about the beneficial and adverse effects of technology is easily made. In Seymour (1999, 2000) it is shown how difficult this might be in the medical setting and what kind of 'negotiation' it might take before reaching a decision. Moreover, in Seymour's (2000) account it would seem evident that medical staff are reluctant to talk about patients' lives in terms of quality of life or good life; instead they focus on the 'natural' limitations or end of biological life.

Hence, even if Callahan is right in claiming that technology has brought us, together with longer lives, worse health, slower deaths, longer illnesses – these longer lives might still, on the whole, be worthwhile lives to live and hence worth the price. However, we might question whether Callahan is right in his claims about the detrimental effects of technology. Even if technology and medicine will not be able to cure all conditions people might end up with, the development seems to move in the direction of making it easier for people to live and die with those conditions (Seymour 1999, 2000; Seymour et al. 2002). Following this, it might not be too much technology and medicine that is the problem but too little, and importantly the users of technology and medicine have confused life per se with worthwhile life. On the other hand, if we accept that worthwhile life is not coextensive with biological life, we would have to accept that it might sometimes be better to die before life is biologically over. (Perhaps even actively end life at that time, something that Callahan does not seem to accept, since he strongly opposes euthanasia.)

Even if technology is not generally detrimental to a good timing of death or even beneficial to such timing, it might still be problematic in making the context of dying and death bad (or worse). In the following, seven suggestions for why technology or machines might have negative effects on the context of death are explored: (a) machines will preclude us from being physically independent; (b) machines will preclude the dying person from being the focus of attention of care personnel; (c) machines will make dying and death less peaceful; (d) machines will make the environement of dying and death less familiar; (e) machines will make dying and death less beautiful or aesthetically becoming; (f) machines will make death less natural; (g) machines will make the dying person lose control over his or her dying and death.

Technology and physical independence

Will the fact that our lives are sustained by machines or that we are connected to machines restrict our physical independence? Obviously yes, we might say. If we compare this with being in full health and with all of our powers and abilities intact, being machine-sustained will, in some ways (continually or intermittently) and in most cases, have a certain restricting effect on our physical independence.

However, there are machines that will make us more physically independent in cases when warranted: take, for example, a pacemaker, which, in aiding a bad heart, enables you to move about more freely. Moreover, when we are dying, these machines might not make much (negative) difference to our physical independence, since not using them would imply that we would be either dead or bedridden. Hence, even if the machine makes us physically restricted, the alternatives at hand might not actually make us more physically independent. Moreover, we might agree that it is better to be physically independent than physically restricted, but not agree that physical restriction makes a life not worth living. That is, physical independence is obviously not all there is to a worthwhile life.

Could we interpret Callahan to mean something stronger by being physically independent, i.e. as having a physique that is self-sufficient and not dependent on anything outside oneself? However, since we obviously are dependent on things outside ourselves (for example, food and drink) we must restrict this idea to dependency on machines. Consequently, if we need a pacemaker and ignore all effects of having to use a pacemaker (good or bad), we would be worse off for being sustained by such a device.

Now, we might agree that it is *ceteris paribus* better to have one's own heart beating away on its own rather than a mechanical device aiding it to do so and still not agree that we cannot benefit from such a device when in a less than ideal situation. When dying I would say we are in a less than ideal situation where mechanical devices might be our best option to achieve as good a life as possible. However, the bad effects of these mechanical devices will obviously have to be taken into account when judging whether a specific patient would benefit from them or not.

Returning to the former statement, imagine someone with a pacemaker and someone with only their own biological heart living exactly the same lives, doing the same things, experiencing the same things, with the same risks of failing being attached to the pacemaker and the heart. Could we actually claim that the latter is, in any way, better off for having only his or her own heart instead of it being aided by a pacemaker? I must admit I have a weak intuition that they would be better off, but I find no good reasons for why this would be so. Hence, I will have to derive that intuition from the fact that normally the pacemaker does not compare to a well functioning heart and, if it did, there would be no real difference as concerns the value of their respective lives. I return to this below, when discussing the naturalness of technology.

In consequence, machines do not always make us more physically restricted than their alternatives, but often the opposite, and we can still live worthwhile lives while physically restricted. Hence, this is not generally a reason why a technological dying would make us worse off.

Technology as focus of attention

The second suggestion for why technology has a negative effect on the context of dying and death is that it diverts attention from the patient to the machines:

> Call to mind an intensive care unit with monitors blinking and beeping and remember how all eyes (even family members') go to the machine – and away from the patient. It requires effort *not* to watch the monitors. Technology – machines, instruments, drug treatments – like blinkers on a horse, restrict and define and thus simplify the viewpoint.
>
> (Cassell 1991: 22)[11]

Or, in Callahan's words:

> Because of the focus on technological intervention, the human relationships are often neglected, judged less important, more dispensable, than the necessity of high-quality technical work. Machines and lab results and scanners become the center of attention; they replace conversation with the patient.
>
> (Callahan 1993: 41)

To the extent that machines need a lot of monitoring and adjustments this will require time and attention that could have been given to the patient more directly. Hence, there is obviously something to this argument. However, in a sense, it is still time and attention given to the benefit of the patient, even if indirectly, since we might assume that the patient is indeed benefited by these machines.

Even so, what the focus of attention of the care personnel will be seems to depend more on the attitudes of the personnel than on the use of technology. In monitoring the machines we have the opportunity to give the patient some 'personal' time. Moreover, if the personnel tend to lose focus on the patient, the patient would get even less attention if there were no machines to monitor in the room. That is, the machines give them a reason to enter the patient's room. Hence, given a bad attitude from the personnel, the machines might even be instrumental in bringing them into contact with the patient.

Consequently, it is not necessarily the technology in itself but the attitude of the personnel that results in diverted attention, even if technology might be used as an excuse to uphold that attitude. Still, without technology we can easily find other excuses for not attending to the patient, as is my own experience from caring for patients. For example, we might refer to the need to do administrative work, the need to update the casebook of the patient, the need to clean out the washing room or whatever. Moreover, the time and energy consumed by the machines might, on the whole, be worth it given that the patient would benefit from the use of these machines. For some patients technological measures that they can manage on their own might even be instrumental in supporting their privacy, to the extent that it is valued by the patients.

The peacefulness of technology

In the section on peacefulness we distinguished between internal and external peace, where the former is a state of mind and the latter a feature of the surrounding environment. Following this distinction, it was argued that even if internal peace in many cases might need external peace in order to be achieved, this is not necessarily so. Besides, even when external peace might be necessary for internal peace, it is not obvious exactly what characterizes external peace.

Hence, we might experience internal peace in the midst of machines and for some people the machines will be necessary in order to achieve internal peace. Consider a person whose fear of asphyxiation is relieved by being put on a ventilator. For such a person, the machine is necessary in order to achieve internal peace. Moreover, from the perspective of external peace we might claim that even if machines do not fit into the traditional picture of peacefulness as a quiet afternoon in the countryside or a silent sea, it might still be a very peaceful scene with the repetitive, dampened and safe sound from the machines.

In conclusion, machines *per se* do not seem detrimental to a peaceful death, even if the use of machines might sometimes deprive us of such a death. This use is not governed by considerations of what on the whole benefits the dying patient in terms of providing further worthwhile life.

Presumably, to rush a dying patient (at the end stage of dying) to the emergency room and put him on a ventilator and keep him thus for a few more hours or days until he dies would generally not seem to provide him with a peaceful death unless it is warranted by the fear and anguish of the dying person. Normally, there are better ways to keep the anguish and fear of the patient under control if prolongation of life is not of essence.

Technology and familiarity

It might be argued that machines invading the environment of the patient will make this environment less familiar to her and hence also bad for her. Now, it is obvious that an unfamiliar environment might cause distress and insecurity and hence lower the well-being of persons in some cases. We do not know our way around such an environment, we do not feel at ease with what to do or do not know what we *can* do in such an environment and we might experience ourselves as not belonging there or being an intruder.

However, first, these problems might be transient and worth the benefits of new experiences that the unfamiliar environment might bring, and an unfamiliar environment might, given time, turn into a familiar one. Second, a familiar environment might not be less distressing (though for other reasons) and an unfamiliar environment might actually be a relief. Moreover, how we experience an unfamiliar environment will depend on things like our awareness of what is happening, our expectations of this environment and whether we are self-confident or not. That is, if the person fully knows and accepts how being transferred into this new environment with all these machines might benefit him and if he is generally confident about himself, the unfamiliarity with the new environment is likely to cause less or no significant lowering of well-being. It might even cause a rise in well-being by providing him with new hope. Hence, whether the unfamiliarity with technology will be bad for the dying person depends on the condition and desires of this person, which, of course, might make it more problematic for dying persons owing to their weakened condition. However, the transient unfamiliarity with the new technological environment might be worth its price if the patient will benefit from the technology in question.

A related idea is that being dependent on machines will make it difficult for us to die in the place of our own choice. In other words, being dependent on advanced technology in dying might preclude us from dying at home and we might want and have good reasons to die at home. It is familiar, it is where we have spent and chosen to spend most of our time, it is where we find ourselves most comfortable. However, some machines are obviously movable and hence do not preclude us from dying at home. Besides, if we are in need of more advanced technology, we might have to face a choice between a shorter (and perhaps more troublesome) life ending at home and a somewhat longer (and perhaps less troublesome) life ending at a hospital. This will be a difficult choice between conflicting or incompatible values where different people are likely to choose differently and it is not obvious which is generally the better choice.

In conclusion, familiarity with an environment has some benefits (hedonistic, desire fulfilment and objective list benefits). However, it seems that we have reasons to forgo such an environment when the gains of an unfamiliar environment outweigh the cost and, to be sure, technology will occasionally bring such gains.

Technology and aesthetics

Perhaps the problem with machines surrounding the dying person is that death is made ugly. Ariés (1981: especially Chapter 10) talks about the ideal of the beautiful death, where death is not ugly or messy or smelly (an ideal that, to be sure, Ariés himself does not seem to embrace). However, in Ballard it is claimed that death is 'usually a messy, agonizing and tortous experience ... [which] it is wrong to sentimentalize and romanticize' (Ballard 1996: 25).[12] In Widgery (1993: 18) it is claimed that, if anything, death makes people ugly and Lawton (2000) provides vivid pictures of decaying dying bodies in her study. This is not always true: I have seen deaths that are none of the above. However, this is far from admitting that death is generally beautiful (Lawton 2000).

From a hedonistic perspective there might be something to this idea, since people generally take an interest in their outward appearances and want to look as good as possible (even if different people might have very different ideals for what this implies). Most of us find it very awkward and uncomfortable believing we are not at our best; just think of the uneasiness we might feel when we believe there is a smell emanating from us. Hence, most people are likely to suffer from the messiness, smell and ugliness that dying might result in (Lawton 2000). In effect, it will in many cases make for a better death to try to care for appearances even in dying and death. However, when it concerns messiness and smell, being connected to a machine or medical device might be one way to gain control over those things and avoid them to some degree. At the least, the machines do not seem to make things more messy or smelly.

So we are left with the idea that machines will make death ugly in the sense of making dying and death of less aesthetic value. In other words, machines will ruin the possibly beautiful picture of death. First, even if death is sometimes portrayed as beautiful and some deaths might even be beautiful according to some aesthetic ideal, generally, I would say they are not. However, even if we admit death to have the potential to be beautiful, would

machines in any way make them less beautiful? Generally, we might consider machines to be ugly and perhaps they often are, but on the other hand
there are also nicely designed machines that might fit into traditionally beautiful or aesthetically rewarding scenery. So, perhaps, we could retain the
beauty of death if the medical machines and devices were better designed.
The absurdity of such a suggestion is that it would seem to indicate that it is
not the beauty of death that will be compromised by the machines. If anything it is the naturalness of death that will be compromised (and the natural
might, in many cases, be thought to be beautiful, at least in a nature-loving
country like Sweden).

Technology and the natural

It is sometimes argued that the use of technology in dying and death will
make these events unnatural or artificial (see Seymour 1999, 2000 for a
discussion of such ideas). Another idea about technology and naturality is
that technology will give us the impression that death is not a natural part of
our lives, but that we can control dying and death. Kübler-Ross (1969: 9)
expresses the latter idea in the following way:

> Is our concentration on equipment, on blood pressure, our desperate
> attempt to deny the impending death which is so frightening and dis-
> comforting to us that we displace all our knowledge onto machines,
> since they are less close us than the suffering face of another human
> being which would remind us once more of our lack of omnipotence,
> our own limits and failures, and last but not least, perhaps our own
> mortality?

Starting with the first idea and following Richard W. Momeyer (1988: 53–8)
we might list six different uses of 'natural': (a) the scientific (or biological),
meaning that something is natural to the extent that it is in line with the laws
of nature; (b) the statistical, meaning that something is natural to the extent
that it is the average occurence of the thing in question; (c) the anthropo-
logical, meaning that something is natural to the extent that it is not man-
made or man-influenced; (d) the conventional, meaning that something is
natural to the extent that it is familiar to us; (e) the theological, meaning that
something is natural to the extent that it is in accordance with God's will; (f)
the evaluative, meaning simply that something is natural when it is morally
correct or good.

The sixth meaning is exactly what is disputed here and we would get a
circular argument if we claimed that technology is bad since it is unnatural
(meaning that it is bad). The fifth meaning will be ignored in this context because of our secular approach, but it is difficult to see why God
would resist technology *per se*. According to the first meaning, technology

would most certainly qualify as natural because it has to 'obey' the laws of nature. Following the second meaning, technology would also qualify as natural (at least in our Western context) since technology is part and parcel of death and dying nowadays (Seymour 2000). As shown by Seymour (2000), technology being seen as natural in this sense might make it rather confusing and difficult to argue against the use of technology on behalf of a natural death; and in Seymour (1999) it is evident that technology is sometimes viewed as something that actually makes for what is seen as a natural death.

Hence, we are left with meanings (c) and (d) as being relevant in this context. Technology and machines are obviously artefacts and hence a death surrounded by machines would be more artificial than a death that is not thus surrounded. On the other hand, beds, sheets and walls are also artefacts and artificial. The same goes for pain-relievers and other medicines and I am fairly sure that the presence of these artefacts is not generally viewed as making death worse (even if more artificial). As mentioned before, a study by Seymour *et al.* (2002) showed that people welcome technology put to a symptom-relieving use. So what is it about machines that might be so problematic?

We are left with the idea that we are normally not connected to machines in our daily life and that we want the context of death to be as close as possible to normal life, for the reason that what is normal is also familiar to us. It has been argued above that we might generally benefit from what is familiar to us. However, as far as the value of dying and death is concerned this only goes part of the way, since most of us would accept deviations from normality and what is familiar to us if we gain something important from such deviations. For example, to go into a hospital and get surgery is presumably not part of what is normal for most people. Still, we find it good (and I would say it is good) due to the benefits we gain from such a deviation. The same would seem to be applicable here. If the gains of being attached to a machine are great enough we have reason to accept it, even if it is a deviation from what is normal to us (and as such unnatural according to the fourth alternative above). To be sure, if being on a ventilator when death is approaching will relieve us of our fear of asphyxiation, this is presumably important enough to warrant a deviation from what is normal to us. On the other hand, in other cases such deviations will not be warranted, since the gains are not great enough and hence to maintain dying and death as close as possible to what is normal (to the particular person) would benefit the dying person more. Hence, even if we often might be best benefited by what is normal to us, there are obviously exceptions and since dying and death is not normal to us (in the sense of something we face often) we have reasons to accept deviations from normality.

Let us also take a look at the idea that technology gives us the wrong impression about being able to control and manage death. It is obvious that technology actually gives us means to control and manage dying and death (even if not fully, in the sense of abolishing it). Arguably, ventilators, infusion pumps, pacemakers and dialysis machines enable us to control and manage both the features of dying and the timing of death to a large extent. Still, technology has not brought us to the point where we fully control and manage dying and death and if the use of technology gives us such an impression, we are obviously fooled by it. However, it is not as obviously true that technology and medicine will not bring us to that point. In other words, if our present use of technology gives us hope to abolish dying and death in the future this might be neither a hope in vain nor a bad hope.

We might distinguish between three different interpretations of the idea that death is a natural part of our lives: (a) it is good that death ends the lives of humans; (b) it is a fact, given the present state of the world, that death ends the lives of humans; (c) it is a necessary fact that death will end the lives of humans.

The second interpretation is obviously true. However, this interpretation has no normative implications in terms of it being good or bad that death ends our lives and, moreover, it does not make any claims about whether the state of the world can change or not. In other words, to say that death is a natural part of life in this sense would have no implications for whether it is a futile or bad hope that technology will abolish death.

The third interpretation, if true, would imply that it is a futile hope (even if not necessarily a bad one) that technology will abolish death. However, this interpretation does not seem obviously true, since it is possible to imagine a world in which creatures with basically the same constitution as us do not die. That is to say, since something causes us to die (fatal illnesses or the wearing down of our organism) there is no principled reason why these causes could not be removed (even if it might never happen due to the complexity of the human being). Consequently, the hope that technology might abolish death (or at least postpone it for a very long time) is not totally futile, even if presumably a long shot. Researchers do, however, claim that it will be possible within a foreseeable future (for example, Bova 1998).

However, from the first interpretation it would be bad for us if we abolished death and dying. Hence, it might be bad for us if technology gives us the wrong impression about the overall value of death. In other contexts (Sandman 2001) I have argued that, provided we can lead a life worth living, death will always be bad for us and would be better abolished (or, at least, postponed into the future as far as possible).

In conclusion, if the use of technology makes us question the naturalness of death, this would not generally be a bad idea (even if we, perhaps, should not be overly optimistic about changing the fact that we all die). Here it must be noted that in relation to a particular patient it might indeed be bad to try to control and manage death to the extent that it is futile and/or causes a worsening of that patient's life (as it might very well do, following the discussion on prolongation of life above).

Who controls technology?

The idea about control is also found in the seventh suggestion for why technology might be detrimental to a good death, but here the focus is on who exercises control of dying and death, the person dying or the person managing the technology. That control over death is an important and dominant feature in the modern literature on good dying and death is obvious. In Seale *et al.* (1997) it is argued that much of the concept of good death we find in palliative care is intimately linked to a general idea about control of the trajectory of one's life. In Seymour *et al.* (2002) it is emphasized that the control of symptom management is essential to a good death.

In relation to most technology, as well as to other medical measures, we need training and skill to be able to manage it and the dying person might not be the one best suited for this job. Hence, on the face of it, the dying person would not be in control of the situation when there is a lot of technology involved. However, as indicated, this would seem to go for most medical measures and we should presumably be reluctant to claim that not being in control of these measures would make for a worse death. Instead, to manage what is problematic in dying and death we should allow the most skilled person to deal with these machines and measures.

On the other hand, there is also technology that gives greater control to the dying person; for example, infusion pumps with which the patient can control when to receive another dose of morphine. Most patients would surely consider that an enhancement of control compared to when doctors or nurses administer new doses every fourth hour or so.

This argument focuses on something important to dying persons. In order for the dying person to keep as much control over her dying as possible, care personnel should be careful only to do to what the patient has approved of or decided. In other words, when dying in a context of dependency it is possibly essential to a lot of people that they are able to control their dying. Suffice it here to say that, given that we assign weight to self-determination and the patient's abilities and possibilities to get what they desire, being in control of technology as well as other measures will often be essential to the dying person, even though it would seem enough if what the dying person decides is accorded with and he or she does not need to be able to manage the machines in question.

Summary

Summing up, technology in dying and death might, as in other context, be put to good as well as bad use and is as such value-neutral (see Loewy and Springer Loewy 2000: 134). Hence, the arguments that tried to show technology to be detrimental to a good death *per se* all failed.

There were some arguments against the use of technology, but they could be countered to the extent that the gain of technology outweighs the cost. Not all will end up siding with the opponents of technology. Aneurin Bevan claimed, when he presented the NHS Bill to the British Parliament, that '[I would] rather be kept alive in the efficient if cold altruism of a large hospital than expire in a gush of warm sympathy in a small one' (quoted in Clark and Seymour 1999: 69).[13] This could be interpreted as support for access to intensive technological and medical measures. In Callahan (1993: 48) it is admitted that 'when a critical illness is at hand, people most often do want many forms of aggressive medical treatment' (Callahan 1993: 48). However, an obvious problem arises when the use of technology does not have any beneficial effects on the life of the dying person; for example, when technology is used to prolong the biological life of the patient without any beneficial effects or only detrimental effects on the value of this patient's life.

Normative aspects of death and technology

What carers should do will depend on the wishes of the dying person and what seems to be the greatest risk here is if there is a generalized view on the use of technology within palliative care, whether it goes in the direction of resistance to or in the direction of welcoming technology. It is important to view technology as a means to the best possible life for the patient and not to lose focus on the patient and her needs.

Could it be justified to use technology for the sake of close ones, even if the patient does not really benefit from such a use? I see no principled reasons for not doing so. However, we need to have three things in mind. First, technology should in such a case not be detrimental to the patient – but at most neutral to her. Second, a justice constraint will probably in all cases preclude us from using expensive technology this way. Third, a constraint about only using what is scientifically warranted might also preclude us from doing so. Hence, there seems in all (or almost all) cases to be a better alternative to try to convince close ones about the fruitlessness of technology when the patient does not benefit from it.

Here it could be added that the structural situation of care could possibly cause misuse of technology, and this is something we have to be aware of. That is, in a situation of care where the implicit norms tend to favour technological activities before other measures, we should be more careful about evaluating the use of technology in the particular case. On the other hand, it is also a problem if the structural situation supports the opposing norm, about not using technology.

Conclusions and relevance to palliative care

In this chapter we have discussed what should characterize the environment of death, whether it should be peaceful or not, whether there should be people present or not, whether we should use technology or not.

In relation to a peaceful environment we distinguished between external and internal peacefulness and it was argued that even if we find some support for the fact that dying people might be more sensitive to noise, it was not obvious that external peacefulness would benefit all dying people. It might instead be interpreted as if life is already over. Hence, even if internal peacefulness would benefit all or most dying people, external peacefulness might not always be the way to achieve internal peacefulness. This is relevant to palliative care to the extent that palliative units or wards tend to be characterized by an external peacefulness not always beneficial to the dying patients, and in my own experience they do tend to be.

In relation to people being present at death it was argued that most people will benefit from being individually acknowledged as important by people close to us, and being present when someone is dying is a way to acknowledge the dying person thus. Still, we found a few reasons for why a dying person might not want to have anyone close present in dying and some reasons for why a professional carer might not be an alternative when the dying person has no close ones to attend her in dying and death. To enable close ones to be present when a person is dying is hence important to palliative care, especially if we want to postpone the social death of the person. However, once again it will be important not to end up with the conclusion that all dying people will benefit from having their close ones present or, if that is not possible, that professional carers are an alternative. They might not be an attractive alternative in the eyes of the dying person.

In relation to technology it was argued that resistance against technology *per se* did not have any strong support. The conclusion was that technology can both benefit and be detrimental to the dying person, depending on how we use it and how we value the life of the dying patient. This not so surprising conclusion is relevant to palliative care, because of the ongoing discussion of medicalization of palliative care and a certain resistance towards this use of advanced technology or medical measures within palliative care.

In effect, once again we find that the environment of a good dying or death could have a number of different characteristics depending on the circumstances and the values of the dying person, even if it is likely that having close ones present in dying will benefit most dying people.

Notes

1 See Saunders and Baines (1983), McNamara *et al.* (1994), Ottoson (in Beck-Friis and Strang 1995), Roy and MacDonald (in Doyle *et al.* 1998), Loewy and Springer Loewy (2000) and Janssens (2001).
2 E. Karlsson, 'Det här skulle vara extremt ovanligt i en svensk familj'. En etnologisk studie om föreställningar krin g etnicitet vid vård i livets slutskede i det egna hemmet. ('This would be extremely unusual in a Swedish family'. An ethnological study of views on ethnicity in home care at the end of life), unpublished manuscript.
3 I have personal experience of working in a hospice situated at one end of a corridor, with an ordinary elderly home situated at the other end. People died at both ends of the corridor, but the environment at the hospice end was more externally peaceful and lacked much of the humorous jargon of the other end. I found this problematic, but the patients might not have shared my views on this.
4 See, for example, Dunstan (1978), Elias (1985), Nuland (1993), Hanratty and Higginson (1994), Brattgård (in Beck-Friis and Strang 1995) and SOU (2001).
5 See Elias (1985) for a discussion of this.
6 See also Kübler-Ross (1974).
7 See Fredriksson-Örndahl *et al.* (1987), McNamara *et al.* (1994), Mitchell (1997) and Janssens (2001).
8 See Twycross (1995) and Beck-Friis and Strang (1995, 1999).
9 See, for example, Clark and Seymour (1999).
10 See also Loewy and Springer Loewy (2000: 2).
11 See also Kübler-Ross (1969: 8).
12 See also Nuland (1993).
13 See also McNamara *et al.* (1994).

7 | Ideas about good dying within palliative care

Now that we have discussed several ideas on what makes for a good dying and death and generally reached the conclusion that we might almost always find reasons to die in a way contrary to these ideas, it is time to say something about the possible role such ideas should play within palliative care.

In Clark and Seymour (1999: 79) it is claimed that: 'Hospice and palliative care has, it might be argued, become synonymous with "good death".'[1] Admitting to the fact that ideas on good dying and death play a role within palliative care, there are different roles they might play and we might arrive at different conclusions concerning which role they should play.[2] To exemplify, ideas on good dying or death might:

- be part of the overall goals for palliative care and something which one tries to achieve in every single case.

This implies that palliative carers try (and, we hope, succeed) in realizing the idea in relation to every single patient. It also means that we use the idea when evaluating whether the palliative care in question was successful. Hence it functions both operatively and evaluatively.

These ideas might:

- function as rules of thumb for what palliative care should try to achieve in every single case.

This implies that palliative carers try to realize the idea under normal circumstances or in the absence of special reasons, but that there might be cases when it should not be realized.

Finally,

- they might provide alternatives in discussions and decisions about what care to provide in a single case.

This implies that the ideas on good death and dying are found on the list of what *can* contribute to a good death and that might be considered in the case at hand.

If we interpret the talk about good dying and death as just another way to say that palliative care should provide patients with as good a quality of life in dying and death as possible, this is obviously in line with the WHO definition of palliative care and something we might reasonably accept in this context: 'Palliative care improves the quality of life of patients and families who face life-threatening illness' (Sepulveda *et al.* 2002). Hence, we might agree that palliative care should provide patients at the end of life with a good dying and a good death, but we might disagree about what this actually amounts to. In effect, we still need to discuss what role we should give to more specific ideas on good dying and death.

In this context I will assume, with the actual arguments being provided elsewhere (Sandman 2003), that specific ideas on good dying and death should mainly function as alternatives in discussion and decision-making within palliative care, with some exceptions that might, at most, function as rules of thumb; the main reason for this being the difficulty in finding universal support for ideas about good dying or death. That is, even when we consider an idea like dying without suffering, which seems to find strong support, it might be the case that we cannot realize this idea, since it sometimes conflicts with other ideas that might be important to the dying person, such as remaining conscious and lucid.

I find it important to emphasize that they do have a role to play to the extent that we agree upon the overall goal of palliative care being good dying for the patient. That is, to the extent that palliative care has such a goal it is essential that one is able to provide patients with help in arriving at what a good dying and death for them amounts to. This is something that the patients might not be fully clear about and that palliative carers might need to help the patients to arrive at. In this book I have tried to show how we can argue for different standpoints in relation to a good dying. In other words, palliative carers cannot just leave it up to the patients to figure out the best way to die on their own, when the patients ask for and obviously need the help of the carers to do this, even if the carers have to be careful not to exercise undue pressure on the patients or have the ambition 'that patients and families will "come around to our way of thinking"', as a nurse expressed it in McNamara *et al.* (1994: 1505). In the words of Seale (1998), carers should be careful not to exercise symbolic violence on the patients. That is, the patients should, if anything, arrive at what is a good dying and death for *them*, given their opinions, values and circumstances – and respect for patients' autonomy should also make us respect patients who are not willing to arrive at any specific ideas about good dying or good death, or who do not want to spend time pondering the matter of good dying or death. There might be good reasons to view such disinterest as one way to achieve the good death, and it is probably the one I would prefer myself.

Notes

1 As indicated above, 'good death' is often used as a comprehensive concept covering the goodness of the period of dying, the event of death and what happens after death. However, in this context I will mainly talk in terms of good dying.
2 For a more thorough discussion of this see Sandman (2003).

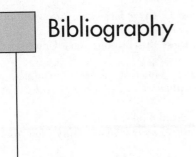

Bibliography

Ågren, M. (1992) Life at 85: a study of life experiences and adjustment of the oldest old. Doctoral dissertation, Institutionen för Geriatrik, Göteborg universitet.

Ågren, M. (1995) En dag i taget: en rapport om livet vid 92 års ålder. Rapport, Institutet för gerontologi i Jönköping, 0282–0927; 75.

Ahlbäck, S., Almqvist, I., Gustavsson, P., Hed, M.-B., Nordqvist-Ericsson, G.-B. and Rask-Carlsson, M. (1998) Handbok för anhöriga – att vårda svårt sjuka och döende i hemmet. Luleå: Vårdcentralerna.

Alston, W. P. (1967) Pleasure, in P. Edwards (ed.) The Encyclopedia of Philosophy. London: Macmillan.

Ariés, P. (1974) Western Attitudes towards Death. Baltimore: Johns Hopkins University Press.

Ariés, P. (1981) The Hour of Our Death. New York: Alfred A. Knopf.

Badham, P. (1996) Theology and the case for euthanasia, in P. Badham and P. Ballard (eds) Facing Death. Cardiff: University of Wales Press.

Ballard, P. (1996) Intimations of mortality: some sociological considerations, in P. Badham and P. Ballard (eds) Facing Death. Cardiff: University of Wales Press.

Bayertz, K. (1996) Human dignity: philosophical origin and scientific erosion of the idea, in K. Bayertz (ed.) Sanctity of Life and Human Dignity. Dordrecht: Kluwer.

Beaty, N. L. (1970) The Craft of Dying: A Study in the Literary Tradition of the Ars Moriendi in England. New Haven, CT: Yale Studies in English.

Beck-Friis, B. (1990) Vård i livets slutskede. Underlag till vårdprogram. Malmö: Malmö utbildningsproduktion.

Beck-Friis, B. and Strang, P. (eds) (1995) Palliativ medicin (Palliative Medicine). Stockholm: Liber.

Beck-Friis, B. and Strang, P. (eds) (1999) Palliativ medicin (Palliative Medicine, 2nd edn). Stockholm: Liber.

Bova, B. (1998) *Immortality. How Science Is Extending Your Life-span and Changing the World*. New York: Avon Books.

Brülde, B. (1998) The human good. Doctoral dissertation, Acta Universitatis Gothoburgensis, Göteborg.

Brülde, B. (2003) Lindrat lidande som den palliativa vårdens huvudmål, in L. Sandman and S. Woods (eds) *God palliativ vård – etiska och filosofiska aspekter*. Lund: Studentlitteratur.

Byock, I. (1997) *Dying Well*. New York: Riverhead Books.

Callahan, D. (1993) *The Troubled Dream of Life. Living with Mortality*. New York: Simon & Schuster.

Cassell, E. J. (1991) *The Nature of Suffering*. Oxford: Oxford University Press.

Clark, D. and Seymour, J. (1999) *Reflections on Palliative Care*. Buckingham: Open University Press.

Clark, J. (2003) Patient centred death. *British Medical Journal*, 327, 174–5

Daniel, J. (1996) Dying and living: philosophical considerations, in P. Badham and P. Ballard (eds) *Facing Death*. Cardiff: University of Wales Press.

De Marinis, V. (1998) *Tvärkulturell vård i livets slutskede – att möta äldre personer med invandrarbakgrund*. Lund: Studentlitteratur.

Doyle, D., Hanks, G. W. C. and MacDonald, N. (1998) *Oxford Textbook of Palliative Medicine*, 2nd edn. Oxford: Oxford University Press.

Dunstan, G. R. (1978) Our duties towards the dying, in C. M. Saunders (ed.) *The Management of Terminal Disease*. London: Edward Arnold.

Dworkin, R. (1993) *Life's Dominion*. London: HarperCollins.

Edgar, A. (1996a) Measuring the quality of life, in P. Badham and P. Ballard (eds) *Facing Death*. Cardiff: University of Wales Press.

Edgar, A. (1996b) Death in our understanding of life, in P. Badham and P. Ballard (eds) *Facing Death*. Cardiff: University of Wales Press.

Edvardson, C. (1984) Rätt att dö värdigt på sina egna villkor, in *Långvård och vårdkultur*. Göteborg: SvD förlag.

Elias, N. (1985) *The Loneliness of the Dying*. Oxford: Blackwell.

Ellingson, S. and Fuller, J. D. (1998) A good death? Finding a balance between the interests of patients and caregivers. *Generations*, 98(3), 87–92.

Feigenberg, L. (1977) *Terminalvård – En metod för psykologisk vård av döende cancerpatienter*. Lund: LiberLäromedel.

Feigenberg, L. (1979) *Döden i sjukvården*. Stockholm: SFPHs monografiserie nr 3.

Feldman, F. (1992) *Confrontations with the Reaper*. New York: Oxford University Press.

Field, D. (1996) Awareness and modern dying. *Mortality*, 1(3), 255–65.

Field, D. and Copp, G. (1999) Communication and awareness about dying in the 1990s. *Palliative Medicine*, 13, 459–68.

Finch, J. (1995) Responsibilities, obligations and commitments, in I. Allen and E. Perkins (eds) *The Future of Family Care for Older People*. London: HMSO.

Finlay, I. (1996) Ethical decision-making in palliative care, in P. Badham and P. Ballard (eds) *Facing Death*. Cardiff: University of Wales Press.

Firth, S. (1993) Approaches to death in Hindu and Sikh communities in Britain, in D. Dickenson and M. Johnson (eds) *Death, Dying and Bereavement*. London: Sage.

Frankl, V. E. (1963) *Man's Search for Meaning*. New York: Simon & Schuster.

Fredriksson-Örndahl, M., Kide, P. and Skinnstad, S. (1987) *Vård i livets slutskede – vårdprogram*. Malmö: Utbildningsproduktion.

Froggatt, K. (1997) Rites of passage and the hospice culture. *Mortality*, 2(2), 123–37.

Furley, D. J. (1986) Nothing to us?, in M. Schofield and G. Striker (eds) *The Norms of Nature*. Cambridge: Cambridge University Press.

Glaser, B. G. and Strauss, A. L. (1965) *Awareness of Dying*. Chicago: Aldine.

Glover, J. (1977) *Causing Death and Saving Lives*. London: Penguin.

Goffman, E. (1967) *Interaction Ritual*. New York: Doubleday Anchor.

Gordijn, B. and Janssens, R. (2000) The prevention of euthanasia through palliative care: new developments in the Netherlands. *Patient Education and Counselling*, 41, 35–46.

Gorer, G. (1955) The pornography of death. *Encounter*, 5(4), 49–52.

Griffin, J. (1986) *Well-being: Its Meaning, Measurement and Moral Importance*. Oxford: Clarendon Press.

Griffin, J. (1996) *Value Judgement. Improving on Ethical Beliefs*. Oxford: Clarendon Press.

Hagerfors, L. (2003) Längta hem. Om ett missionärsbarn i Kongo. Stockholm: Norstedts.

Hanratty, J. F. and Higginson, I. (1994) *Palliative Care in Terminal Illness*, 2nd edn. Oxford: Radcliffe Medical Press.

Harris, J. (1985) *The Value of Life*. London: Routledge & Kegan Paul.

Harris, J. (2000) Intimations of immortality. *Science*, 288(5463), 59.

Honeybun, J., Johnson, M. and Tookman, A. (1992) The impact of a patient death on fellow hospice patients. *British Journal of Medical Psychology*, 65, 67–72.

Janssens, R. (2001) *Palliative Care. Concepts and Ethics*. Nijmegen: Nijmegen University Press.

Kamm, F. (1993) *Morality, Mortality*. New York: Oxford University Press.

Kolnai, A. (1995) Dignity, in R. S. Dillon (ed.) *Dignity, Character, and Self-respect*. New York: Routledge.

Kübler-Ross, E. (1969) *On Death and Dying*. London: Macmillan.

Kübler-Ross, E. (1974) *Questions and Answers on Death and Dying*. New York: Ross Medical Associates.

Lantz, G. (1992) *Vårdetik. Berättelsen om Arthur*. Falun: Almqvist & Wiksell.

Lantz, G. (2003) Vårdteologi och palliativ vård, in L. Sandman and S. Woods (eds) *God palliativ vård – etiska och filosofiska aspekter*. Lund: Studentlitteratur.

Larsson, R. (1984) *En hand att hålla i – en appell för bättre vård i livets slutskede*. Stockholm: Bonnierfakta.

Lawton, J. (2000) *The Dying Process. Patients' Experiences of Palliative Care*. London: Routledge.

Lehtinen, U.-L. (1998) Underdog shame. Philosophical essays on women's internalization of inferiority. Doctoral dissertation, Department of Philosophy, University of Gothenburg.

Lindqvist, K. (1980) *Att vara med döende*. Stockholm: Liber Läromedel.

Loewy, E. H. and Springer Loewy, R. (2000) *The Ethics of Terminal Care. Orchestrating the End of Life*. New York: Kluwer Academic/Plenum.

Lofland, L. H. (1978) *The Craft of Dying: The Modern Face of Death.* Beverly Hills, CA: Sage.

Longaker, C. (1996) *Facing Death and Finding Hope. A Guide to the Emotional and Spiritual Care of the Dying.* New York: Doubleday.

McNamara, B., Waddell, C. and Colvin, M. (1994) The institutionalization of the good death. *Social Science and Medicine,* 39(11), 1501–8.

Maguire, P. and Faulkner, A. (1993) Communicating with cancer patients. 2: Handling uncertainty, collusion and denial, in D. Dickenson and M. Johnson (eds) *Death, Dying and Bereavement.* London: Sage.

Mitchell, D. R. (1997) The good death: three promises to make at the bedside. *Geriatrics,* 52(8), 91–3.

Momeyer, R. W. (1988) *Confronting Death.* Bloomington: Indiana University Press.

Noll, P. (1985) *Den utmätta tiden (Diktate über Sterben und Tod mit Totenrede von Max Frisch).* Stockholm: Brombergs Bokförlag.

Nordenfelt, L. (2003) Dignity of the elderly: an introduction. *Medicine, Health Care and Philosophy,* 6, 99–101.

Nozick, R. (1989) *The Examined Life: Philosophical Meditations.* New York: Touchstone, Simon & Schuster.

Nuland, S. B. (1993) *How We Die.* New York: Alfred A. Knopf.

Nussbaum, M. C. (1994) *The Therapy of Desire. Theory and Practice in Hellenistic Ethics.* Princeton, NJ: Princeton University Press.

O'Connor, M. C. (1942) *The Art of Dying Well: The Development of the Ars Moriendi.* New York: Columbia University Press.

Öhlén, J. (2000) Att vara i en fristad – berättelser om lindrat lidande inom palliativ vård. Doctoral dissertation, Institutionen för vårdpedagogik, Göteborg.

Parfit, D. (1984) *Reasons and Persons.* Oxford: Clarendon Press.

Parkes, C. M. (1978) Psychological aspects, in C. M. Saunders (ed.) *The Management of Terminal Disease.* London: Edward Arnold.

Payne, S., Hillier, R., Langley-Evans, A. and Roberts, T. (1996) Impact of witnessing death on hospice patients. *Social Science Medicine,* 43(12), 1785–94.

Qvarnström, U. (1993) *Vår död.* Arlöv: Almqvist & Wiksell.

Randall, F. and Downie, R. S. (1996) *Palliative Care Ethics. A Good Companion.* Oxford: Oxford University Press.

Rinell-Hermansson, A. (1990) Det sista året – Omsorg och vård i livets slutskede. Doctoral dissertation, Acta Universaliensis, Uppsala.

Samson Katz, J. (1993) Jewish perspectives on death, dying and bereavement, in D. Dickenson and M. Johnson (eds) *Death, Dying and Bereavement.* London: Sage.

Sandman, L. (2001) A good death: on the value of death and dying. Doctoral dissertation, Acta Universitatis Gothoburgensis, Göteborg.

Sandman, L. (2002) What's the use of human dignity within palliative care? *Nursing Philosophy,* 3, 177–81.

Sandman, L. (2003) Vilken roll bör idéer om en god död spela i palliativ vård?, in L. Sandman and S. Woods (eds) *Palliativ vård – etiska och filosofiska aspekter.* Lund: Studentlitteratur.

Sandman, L. (2004) On the autonomy turf. Assessing the value of autonomy to patients. *Medicine, Health-Care and Philosophy,* in press.

Saunders, C. M. (1978a) Appropriate treatment and dignified death, in C. M. Saunders (ed.) *The Management of Terminal Disease.* London: Edward Arnold.

Saunders, C. M. (1978b) The philosophy of terminal care, in C. M. Saunders (ed.) *The Management of Terminal Disease.* London: Edward Arnold.

Saunders C. M. and Baines M. (1983) *Living with Dying. The Management of Terminal Disease.* Oxford: Oxford University Press.

Saunders, Y., Ross, J. R. and Riley, J. (2003) Planning for a good death: responding to unexpected events. *British Medical Journal,* 327, 204–6.

Sen, A. (1992) *Inequality Re-examined.* Oxford: Clarendon Press.

Seale, C. (1998) *Constructing Death. The Sociology of Dying and Bereavement.* Cambridge: Cambridge University Press.

Seale, C. (2000) Changing patterns of death and dying. *Social Science and Medicine,* 51, 917–30.

Seale, C., Addington-Hall, J. and McCarthy, M. (1997) Awareness of dying: prevalence, causes and consequences. *Social Science Medicine,* 45(3), 477–84.

Sepulveda, C., Marlin, A., Yoshida, T. and Ullrich, A. (2002) Palliative care: the World Health Organization's global perspective. *Journal of Pain and Symptom Management,* 24(2), 91–6.

Seymour, J. E. (1999) Revisiting medicalisation and 'natural' death. *Social Science and Medicine,* 49, 691–704.

Seymour, J. E. (2000) Negotiation natural death in intensive care. *Social Science and Medicine,* 51, 1241–52.

Seymour, J. E., Bellamy, G., Gott, M., Ahmedzai, S. H. and Clark, D. (2002) Good deaths, bad deaths: older people's assessments of the risks and benefits of morphine and terminal sedation in end-of-life care. *Health, Risk and Society,* 4(3), 287–303.

Singer, I. (1996) *The Creation of Value.* Baltimore: Johns Hopkins University Press.

Smart, J. J. C. and Williams, B. (1973) *Utilitarianism: For and Against.* Cambridge: Cambridge University Press.

Smith, R. (2000) A good death. An important aim for health services and for us all. *British Medical Journal,* 320, 130–1.

SOU (1979) *I livets slutskede. Huvudbetänkande från utredningen rörande frågor beträffande sjukvård i livets slutskede.* Stockholm: SLS, Socialdepartementet.

SOU (2001) *Döden angår oss alla. Värdig vård vid livets slut.* Stockholm: Fritzes Offentliga Publikationer.

Sudnow, D. (1967) *Passing On: The Social Organization of Dying.* Englewood Cliffs, NJ: Prentice Hall.

Swarte, N. B., van der Lee, M., van der Bom, J. G., van den Bout, J. and Heintz, A. P. M. (2003) Effects of euthanasia on the bereaved family and friends: a cross sectional study. *British Medical Journal,* 327, 189–92.

Tännsjö, T. (1998a) *Hedonistic Utilitarianism.* Edinburgh: Edinburgh University Press.

Tännsjö, T. (1998b) *Vårdetik.* Stockholm: Thales.

Tännsjö, T. (2003) Terminal sedering, ett alternative i god palliativ vård?, in L. Sandman and S. Woods (eds) *God palliativ vård – etiska och filosofiska aspekter.* Lund: Studentlitteratur.

Ternestedt, B.-M. (1994) *Ett hospice växer fram – från idé till verklighet.* Örebro: Örebro Läns Landsting.

Ternestedt, B.-M. (1998) *Livet pågår! Om vård av döende*. Stockholm: Vårdförbundet.

Thomas, D. (1952) *The Collected Poems*. New York: New Directions.

Tolstoy, L. (1974) *Ivan Iljitjs död, Familjelycka, Herre och dräng*. Uddevalla: Forum.

Twycross, R. (1995) *Introducing Palliative Care*. Oxford: Radcliffe Medical Press.

Walter, T. (1993) Modern death: taboo or not taboo?, in D. Dickenson and M. Johnson (eds) *Death, Dying and Bereavement*. London: Sage.

Walter, T. (1994) *The Revival of Death*. London: Routledge.

Walter, T. (2003) Historical and cultural variants on the good death. *British Medical Journal*, 327, 218–20.

Weisman, A. D. (1972) *On Dying and Denying: A Psychiatric Study of Terminality*. New York: Behavioral Publications.

Weisman, A. D. (1973) Coping with untimely death. *Psychiatry*, 36(4).

Weisman, A. D. (1974) *The Realization of Death. A Guide for the Psychological Autopsy*. New York: Jason Aronson.

Weisman, A. D. and Hackett, T. P. (1961) Predilection to death. Death and dying as a psychiatric problem. *Psychosomatic Medicine*, 23, 232–56.

Widgery, D. (1993) Not going gently, in D. Dickenson and M. Johnson (eds) *Death, Dying and Bereavement*. London: Sage.

World Health Organization (1990) *Cancer Pain Relief and Palliative Care*. Technical Report Series No. 804. Geneva: World Health Organization.

Index

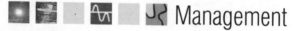
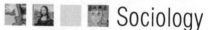
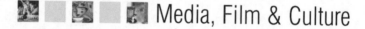
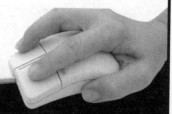
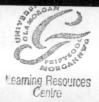

Learning Resources
Centre